EFFECTIVE W] HEALTHCARE PI

This new edition of *Effective Writing for Healthcare Professionals: A Pocket Guide to Getting Published* is an invaluable insider's guide to publishing, providing tips and advice for time-poor professionals working in the healthcare sector.

But how do you get published? Where do you start? How do you know if your writing is good enough, and what can you learn to make it better? Offering an accessible guide to the key issues, this is the perfect book for those who have busy working lives and find the process of writing challenging. It covers issues ranging from getting started to the winning habits of successful authors; from the rights and responsibilities of authors to how to get noticed. This new edition has been updated to include guidance on publishing norms, collaborative digital platforms, social media, and the impact of the COVID-19 pandemic on publishing trends.

Written by a best-selling academic author, this is an essential resource for novice writers and healthcare providers interested in publishing their work.

Megan-Jane Johnstone AO is a retired professor of nursing who now writes as an independent scholar. She is the author of several books including *Alzheimer's Disease, Media Representations and the Politics of Euthanasia*, and *Bioethics: A Nursing Perspective*.

EFFECTIVE WRITING FOR HEALTHCARE PROFESSIONALS

A POCKET GUIDE TO GETTING PUBLISHED

SECOND EDITION

MEGAN-JANE JOHNSTONE

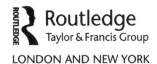

Routledge
Taylor & Francis Group

LONDON AND NEW YORK

Designed cover image: Getty Images

Second edition published 2024
by Routledge
4 Park Square, Milton Park, Abingdon, Oxon, OX14 4RN

and by Routledge
605 Third Avenue, New York, NY 10158

Routledge is an imprint of the Taylor & Francis Group, an informa business

First edition published by Allen & Unwin 2004

British Library Cataloguing-in-Publication Data
A catalogue record for this book is available from the British Library

Library of Congress Cataloging-in-Publication Data
Names: Johnstone, Megan-Jane, author.
Title: Effective writing for healthcare professionals : a pocket guide to getting published / Megan-Jane Johnstone.
Description: Second edition. | Milton Park, Abingdon, Oxon ; New York, NY : Routledge, 2024. | Includes bibliographical references and index. | Summary: "This new edition of Effective Writing for Healthcare Professionals is an invaluable insider's guide to publishing, providing tips and advice for time-poor professionals working in the healthcare sector. Written by a best-selling academic author, this is an essential resource for novice writers and healthcare providers interested in publishing their work"— Provided by publisher.
Identifiers: LCCN 2023022145 | ISBN 9781032537009 (hardback) | ISBN 9781032537023 (paperback) | ISBN 9781003413226 (ebook)
Subjects: LCSH: Medical writing—Handbooks, manuals, etc.
Classification: LCC R119 .J58 2024 | DDC 808.06/661—dc23/eng/20230722
LC record available at https://lccn.loc.gov/2023022145

ISBN: 978-1-032-53700-9 (hbk)
ISBN: 978-1-032-53702-3 (pbk)
ISBN: 978-1-003-41322-6 (ebk)

DOI: 10.4324/9781003413226

Typeset in Adobe Garamond Pro
by Apex CoVantage, LLC

To Helen Fahey (b. 1930), and the generation of busy healthcare providers she represents who, because of the times they lived in, never had the opportunity to publish their vital experiences so that others may learn.

| CONTENTS

| PREFACE

The idea to write this book and its compilation is a response to the many colleagues, associates, and students who—over the past several years—have asked for advice on how they might begin a writing career and succeed as authors. Healthcare professionals can make a difference to the world in which they live and work by publishing their work in a range of media including professional journals, academic and professional books, reports, social media, weblogs, professional newsletters, and the mass-circulation media. Unfortunately, many would-be writers in the healthcare professions—especially busy direct-care providers and administrators, junior academics with high teaching loads, and students—are often intimidated by the thought of writing and become their own instruments of discouragement. The primary aim of this book is to overturn this 'writing block' and to guide aspiring authors in the healthcare disciplines towards becoming their own mentors and instruments of encouragement and success.

In the chapters to follow information is presented in the hope that it will:

- assist readers to get focused on achieving their professional writing and publication goals
- demonstrate that writing is not just an intellectual event, but a craft, an art, and a science that can be learned and developed
- show how writing and publication is not just about producing scholarly articles and foundational texts, but about having a voice, naming a reality, touching an audience,

developing professional self-understanding, advancing a cause, and transforming the world in which healthcare professionals live and work

- improve understanding of the processes for getting writing published
- highlight the nature and imperatives of upholding publishing norms
- facilitate readers on their journey and transformation from writer to author.

It is further hoped that, upon reading this book, healthcare professionals who have previously felt daunted by the prospect of writing will feel more confident about engaging in the writing process, get their work published, and succeed as authors in their field of practice.

ACKNOWLEDGEMENTS

In writing this book, I have become indebted to a number of people. Foremost among these people are the many busy direct-care providers and administrators who have generously shared with me their stories of 'fears and failures' as aspiring authors and who have encouraged me to write this work. Their stories and aspirations have significantly influenced the nature and content of this book. Acknowledgement and thanks are also due to the publishing team at Routledge/Taylor & Francis. In particular, thanks are due to Russell George (senior editor, public health and allied health) for encouraging me to undertake the project of preparing this second revised edition, Amy Thomson (editorial assistant) for her due diligence and prompt responses to my many queries, Kurt R. Zimmer (copy editor) for his copy editing of the final manuscript before going to press, and Christopher Mathews, Senior Project Manager, for overseeing the final production of this book for publication.

1 | WRITING, PUBLICATION, AND SCHOLARSHIP IN THE HEALTHCARE PROFESSIONS

INTRODUCTION

Healthcare professionals spend many hours of their working day writing. This writing, largely undertaken for reasons of day-to-day professional communication, may take the form of responding to email, compiling client case histories, annotating progress notes, writing letters, and preparing various reports on a range of work-related matters. Some healthcare professionals may also spend many hours writing outside of their usual work time, including writing entries in a reflective practice journal, composing an essay to meet the assessment requirements of a university course, or preparing a presentation for a staff development seminar or professional conference.

Despite the vast amounts of time that healthcare professionals spend writing in the course of their everyday work, few write specifically for the purposes of scholarly publication—even though publication in professional journals and foundational texts can have enormous benefits and rewards. For many healthcare professionals, the day-to-day demands of writing notes, compiling reports, and so on, is a burden and a chore. Thus, any idea that writing for publication could be a pleasant and rewarding experience might appear to be—at best—far-fetched and—at worse—misguided.

WRITING, PUBLICATION, AND SCHOLARSHIP

Being a *writer* is not the same as being a *scholar* (i.e., someone with academic expertise and who is highly motivated to

DOI: 10.4324/9781003413226-1

advance knowledge through in-depth study, research, and publication). This is because 'writing', defined by the *Oxford English Dictionary* (OED) (2023c̲) as the 'action or process of forming or setting down letters, symbols or words on a surface such as paper with a pen, pencil, brush, etc.' (*from Old English wrītan—originally: to scratch runes into bark*) literally involves nothing more than *marking words on paper*. Unless *published*— literally 'made public'—writing per se remains hidden from view and, as such, can have little influence beyond the page upon which it is written.

Publication (and grammatical variations thereof), as indicated previously, may be defined as 'the action of making something publicly known' (*from Latin pūblicāre to make public*) (OED, 2023a). As will be shown later in this book, works can be published using *traditional* modes (e.g., peer-reviewed journals, conference proceedings, and foundational texts) and *non-traditional* modes (e.g., online blogs and other digital and social media platforms) (Acquaviva et al., 2020). *Scholarship*, in turn, relates to the pursuit and dissemination of knowledge and, for the purposes of this discussion, is defined as

> Of, relating to, or characteristic of an educational institution or environment; concerned with the pursuit of research, education, and scholarship; scholarly, educational, intellectual. Of or relating to an academy for the cultivation and promotion of literature, of arts and sciences, or of some particular art or science or branch of these; of or relating to a member of such an academy.
>
> (OED, 2023b̲)

Given these definitions, it is clear that although distinct, the three processes of writing, publication, and scholarship are inextricably linked, noting that one cannot proceed without the other. Using these processes effectively, however, requires learned skills and scholarly competence, a beginning guide to which this book hopes to provide.

THE IMPORTANCE OF WRITING FOR PUBLICATION

There is no doubt that writing for publication and getting a manuscript published is hard work. Nonetheless, publishing can be an extremely rewarding experience on both personal and professional levels. On a personal level, getting a worked published can bring a great deal of personal satisfaction. On a professional level, the rewards of establishing a publication track record can include:

- professional development
- professional kudos and recognition
- career advancement.

In addition to the personal and professional rewards that can be gained by publishing professional works, there are other important professional reasons and imperatives for writing for publication.

Crucial to the development of any profession's unique body of knowledge and practice is the publication of its own distinctive professional scholarship. Further, it is vital that a profession's canon becomes well known to those both within and outside the profession, since this helps to facilitate both self and public scrutiny of the profession's knowledge and practice, as well as the profession's responsibility and accountability to the public. Given these and related considerations, there is room to suggest that the issue of professional scholarship and publishing is an important one for members of the healthcare professions.

THE GREATEST STORIES NEVER TOLD

Healthcare professionals often have a wealth of knowledge and experience that deserves to be—and, as a matter of moral imperative, *ought* to be—'made public': in other words, be *published*. This is especially so in cases when the publication of certain experiences and the knowledge gained from these experiences can provide valuable learning opportunities for others. Despite this, many healthcare professionals do not write for publication or submit work for publication in a professional journal or other publication outlets. This is so even though, today, there are open opportunities to formally publish case reports, case studies, correspondence, essays, opinion articles, and policy briefs in addition to the research and methodology articles in reputable peer-reviewed health professional journals (see, for example, Routledge Article Guidelines, https://routledgeopenresearch.org/for-authors/article-guidelines/).

Several years ago, I was present at an in-house seminar where an experienced clinician gave a heart-rending account of how she had dealt with an ethical dilemma in the intensive-care unit where she worked. Her story involved the care of a man who was estranged from his identical twin brother whom he had not seen for several years. The man's condition was serious, and it was evident that he was dying. Despite being aware of his deteriorating condition, the man was adamant that 'he did not want any contact with his twin brother' and that 'his twin brother was not to be contacted and told about his condition'. Having personally experienced the relationship dynamics between twins in her own family, and feeling intuitively that the man was not making the 'right' choice in the circumstances at hand, the clinician decided to respectfully disagree with her patient's request and to act against his expressed wishes. Recognising that time was running out (the man was not expected to live very long), she immediately set in motion a chain of events that resulted in the estranged brothers being happily reunited and reconciled before the ill brother died. Prior to the ill twin's death, both brothers were insistent that the attending clinician had done the right thing and expressed their deep appreciation for her insights, sensitivity, and actions—especially her decision to go against the ill twin's expressed wishes.

The clinician's story provoked much controversy and discussion among those present. Many were perplexed by the clinician's blatant, albeit considered, disregard of her patient's expressed wishes. Nonetheless, they recognised that they had been privy to a unique learning experience and were unanimous in their response that the clinician should write up her story and get it published—not least because of the valuable learning it offered to others who might find themselves in a similar situation. The clinician responded shyly to this encouragement, stating only that she would think about it. Even though the views and counterviews expressed that day yielded all the ingredients for what promised to be a classic article on the ethics of respecting patients' choices, to this day the clinician has not published her story, or an analysis of it from a bioethics perspective. As a result, others have been deprived of a valuable learning experience. Why?

HURDLES TO PUBLISHING

The clinician's decision not to publish her story and the possible reasons influencing her decision are not unique. Indeed, there are many reasons why members of the healthcare professions—especially busy clinicians and managers—do not publish. Although there is a paucity of current research on this subject, research conducted in the 1990s consistently identified lack of time, confidence (i.e., by aspiring authors in their own ability to write and publish), mentorship, technical support, research funding, motivation, and personal interest in publishing as being the most commonly cited reasons for low publication rates by members of the healthcare professions (McConnell & Paech, 1993; Martin & Birnbrauer, 1996; Marchiori et al., 1998; Roberts, 1996; Turnbull & Roberts, 2002; Wilson & Thomson, 1999). Anecdotal evidence today suggests that these reasons remain salient.

Frontline healthcare providers and managers continue to work in understaffed and high stress environments—a factor that became especially apparent during the COVID-19 pandemic. After a hectic day's work, those on the frontline may feel that they have little energy to *think*, let alone write a research report, a reflective essay, or a commentary on a professional or practice issue. Furthermore, even those who work in academic institutions (and who are *expected* to publish as part of their specified work duties) often find it difficult to meet the performance requirements of their roles. The status quo need not stand, however. It is possible—despite the constraints of work and time—to develop what some authors have called 'a community of scholars' within the healthcare professions and to increase the publication rates within this population (Ramani et al., 2021, p. 966). The question is: where to begin?

Healthcare professionals are already deeply engaged in the processes of writing as a means of purposeful communication in the course of their day-to-day work. The challenge ahead is to extend this writing to a broader range of projects and a broader audience. To achieve this, however, a more 'futuristic' and proactive strategy is required. And although the future cannot be predicted with certainty, a preferred future depicting a writer's highest aspirations can nonetheless be envisaged. Writers can also choose to shape their future according to these aspirations, as opposed to merely allowing themselves to be at the mercy of outside forces and circumstances that may converge to impede their pathways to success. To succeed at this task, however, novice authors need to change the way they think and work, and to *believe that they can succeed*. Accordingly, progressing publishing and scholarship in the healthcare professions rests on aspiring authors:

- clarifying their aspirations and goals as authors in their chosen fields
- stepping back from the hustle and bustle of their daily routines to think about their future and where they want to be
- examining whether their decisions and actions are really (and realistically) directed at pursuing and achieving their publishing aspirations and goals
- recognising that while they cannot predict the future, they can, nevertheless, envisage a preferred future for being a successful author and scholar
- believing that they can succeed.

CONCLUSION

Writing is a core activity in the healthcare professions. Nevertheless, only a select few (e.g., academics and researchers) in these professions write *specifically* for the purpose of publication. There are many reasons why direct-care providers do not publish, including but not limited to a lack of time, a lack of support from employers and peers, and a lack of confidence.

There are many healthcare professionals—both in the past and present—who have felt strongly about something, who have taken huge personal risks to engage in actions that have demonstrably helped others, and/or who have discovered something during the course of their practice that is 'working' to the benefit of either their patients, their co-workers, or their profession—and yet for a variety of reasons have neither written about nor published their vital experiences. This failure to publish—and hence, failure to share with others—the knowledge and insights they have gained in relation to their experience results in lost knowledge, which can have a profound impact on the lives of others—not least those dependent on them for care and/or service.

The primary objective of effective writing and publication in the healthcare disciplines is to make a significant and original contribution of knowledge to the field and to participate productively and influentially in professional conversations that have as their objective:

- questioning and calling into question 'things as they are'
- disseminating information and sharing knowledge that could improve policy and practice
- facilitating self and public scrutiny of a profession and its practice
- fostering professional accountability and responsibility to the public
- generally promoting the development of the discipline and the profession.

EXERCISES

1 Write down your professional goals and aspirations as a writer/author.
2 List what you perceive as being the key obstacles to you achieving your writing/publication goals.
3 Outline what you believe would assist you to overcome the obstacles you have identified in question 2.
4 Talk to a colleague or an associate who has had an article published in a peer-reviewed professional journal

or who has had other works published. Ask them to tell you about their first experience of writing for publication. Ask what motivated them to write, how they got started, and why they think publishing is important. Finally, ask them about what contribution they believe their work has made to their field/profession.

5 Talk to a colleague or an associate who has *not* published anything. Ask them to tell you why they have not published in a professional capacity and what—if anything—would motivate or assist them to write an article for publication in a professional journal.

6 Make a list of issues or ideas you think you would like to write about.

7 Imagine a preferred publishing future for yourself.

REFERENCES

Acquaviva, K. D., Mugele, J., Abadilla, N., Adamson, T., Bernstein, S. L., Bhayani, R. K., . . . Trudell, A. M. (2020). Documenting social media engagement as scholarship: A new model for assessing academic accomplishment for the health professions. *Journal of Medical Internet Research*, *22*(12), e25070. DOI: 10.2196/25070

Marchiori, D. M., Meeker, W., Hawk, C., & Long, C. R. (1998). Research productivity of chiropractic college faculty. *Journal of Manipulative and Physiological Therapeutics*, *21*(1), 8–13.

Martin, P., & Birnbrauer, J. (1996) Introduction to clinical psychology. In *Clinical psychology: Profession and practice in Australia* (pp. 3–20). Macmillan Education AU.

McConnell, E., & Paech, M. (1993). Trends in scholarly nursing literature. *Australian Journal of Advanced Nursing*, *11*(2), 28–32.

Oxford English Dictionary (OED). (2023a, March). *Publication, n. OED online*. Oxford University Press. Retrieved from www.oed.com/view/Entry/154060

Oxford English Dictionary (OED). (2023b, March). *Scholarship, n. OED online.* Oxford University Press. Retrieved from www.oed. com/view/Entry/172495

Oxford English Dictionary (OED). (2023c, March). *Academic, n. and adj. OED online.* Oxford University Press. Retrieved from https://www-oed-com.ezproxy-f.deakin.edu.au/view/Ent ry/880?rskey=FjDPdQ&result=3

Ramani, S., McKimm, J., Findyartini, A., Nadarajah, V. D., Hays, R., Chisolm, M. S., . . . & Wilson, K. W. (2021). Twelve tips for developing a global community of scholars in health professions education. *Medical Teacher, 43*(8), 966–971. DOI: 10.1080/0142159X.2020.1839034

Roberts, K. L. (1996). A snapshot of Australian nursing scholarship 1993–1994. *Collegian, 3*(1), 4–10.

Turnbull, B. J., & Roberts, K. K. (2002). Scholarly productivity: Are nurse academics catching up?. *The Australian Journal of Advanced Nursing, 20*(2), 8–14.

Wilson, N., & Thomson, G. (1999). Content analysis and publication outcomes of projects by public health medicine registrars. *Australian and New Zealand Journal of Public Health, 23*(5), 541–542. DOI: 10.1111/j.1467–842X.1999.tb01315.x

2 | GETTING STARTED

INTRODUCTION

Getting started can sometimes be an intimidating experience, even for the most accomplished of writers. As one experienced writer put it, 'The sight of a blank sheet of paper always intimated me; I felt too discouraged to even try more than a sentence or two' (Bryant, 1999, p. 7). This writer eventually overcame the intimidation she felt at the sight of a blank sheet of paper and is now a successful author and seminar leader who has taught thousands of aspiring writers on the art, craft, and science of writing.

Feeling intimidated by a blank sheet of paper—or a blank computer screen—and feeling daunted by the task of commencing a new work is entirely *normal* and more common than is admitted publicly. Even the award-winning US author Stephen King (who has published 64 novels and sold over 35 million copies of his books) has revealed feeling intimidated when beginning an act of writing. In his memoir, *On Writing*, King reveals

> The scariest moment is always just before you start. After that, things can only get better . . . if you are brave enough to start, you will.
>
> (King, 2000, pp. 218–219)

Not only is feeling intimated 'normal', but it stands as a humble reminder that in many respects all writers—even experienced authors—are 'beginners'. As Scott Edelstein (a US writer, editor and literary agent, and author of *100 Things Every Writer Needs to Know*) explains:

DOI: 10.4324/9781003413226-2

> Every writer starts out as a beginner . . . . All of us remain beginners no matter how much writing experience we may accumulate. After all, each time you start a new piece, you're bringing into existence something that hasn't existed before.
>
> (Edelstein, 1999, p. 6)

The key to overcoming this intimidation, and the frustration and discouragement that inevitably comes with it, is to:

- be clear about what your writing goals are and to focus persistently on achieving them
- get straight down to the business of choosing a topic, deciding your audience, and selecting your publishing outlet
- commence the process of writing
- have courage and persevere, even when seeming to fail.

In regard to the latter, as the UK author J.K. Rowling (author of the famed Harry Potter book series) notes:

> Fear of failure is the saddest reason on earth not to do what you were meant to do. I finally found the courage to start submitting my first book to agents and publishers at a time when I felt a conspicuous failure. Only then did I decide that I was going to try this one thing and that I always suspected I could do, and if it didn't work out, well, I'd faced worse and survived
>
> (Rowling, 2019).

She concludes:

> Ultimately, wouldn't you rather be the person who actually finished the project you're dreaming about, rather than the one who talks about 'always having wanted to'?
>
> (Rowling, 2019)

GETTING FOCUSED ON ACHIEVING YOUR WRITING GOALS

As indicated in Chapter 1, it is important that you clarify your writing aspirations and goals right at the outset of your writing career. This can be achieved by spending a few moments completing a simple self-assessment exercise that requires you to consider and note down:

- your mission as a writer
- your reasons for wanting to write
- what you most wish to achieve with your writing.

In completing your self-assessment, and embarking on your writing career, it is important that you:

- set realistic publishing goals
- are path-orientated
- find a mentor to support you through your journey
- have a sense of your own 'voice'.

Different people will have different mission statements, different reasons for wanting to write, and different aspirations in regard to what precisely it is that they want to write and achieve with their writing. This difference is to be expected and should not be used as a measure for assessing the possible strengths and weaknesses of your own statements. What is important is that *you*, as an aspiring writer, are:

- clear about what it is you want to write and achieve
- determined to achieve your goals
- prepared to take the action and put in the effort necessary to realise your writing aspirations.

When I have facilitated seminars on 'writing for publication', I have asked participants to identify the reasons behind their desire to write. The reasons given have ranged from being deeply personal to profoundly professional and/or political in nature. Reasons commonly cited by seminar participants concerning why they want to write have included:

- to be visible
- so thoughts do not get lost
- to move on
- to prompt others
- to improve/advance ideas/others
- so others can read
- so others can be empowered
- I have something to say
- to find out what I know
- it feels good to order my thoughts on a [computer] screen
- for pleasure
- to alleviate pain/to heal
- to survive
- to make sense
- to inform
- to challenge
- to communicate with others
- to develop as a person
- to develop self-understanding
- to make a difference.

Those who write professionally and who have published extensively (both fiction and non-fiction writers) cite similar reasons for why they write (see, for example Blythe, 1998; hooks, 1999; King, 2000). Another reason cited by successful authors on why they write, is simply that they have a *need* to write. Like artists who 'need' to create art, and musicians who 'need' to create music, some writers simply 'need' to write. When addressing a question about what she most loved about her writing life, J.K. Rowling (discussed earlier) responded, 'It's more of a need than a love' (Rowling, 2019).

Once you have clarified your mission as a writer, the reasons why you want to write, and the goals you wish to achieve, there remains the tasks of choosing and confirming a topic, deciding what approach to take (e.g., whether to write a case study, an opinion article, an essay on the topic chosen, or a research report), identifying your intended audience, and choosing the best platform for getting your work published (e.g., a peer-reviewed journal, an organisation newsletter, a blog). Often these things are decidedly simultaneously, but for the purposes of this discussion, they will be presented chronologically.

CHOOSING A TOPIC

Some of the richest sources of ideas and topics on which to write are your *own* observations and intuitions. Key issues and critical questions can be identified by:

- being observant
- looking for imperfections in things
- noting your own and others' dissatisfaction with things
- searching for causes
- being sensitive to implications
- recognising the opportunities embedded in controversy
- following your interest/curiosity—'following your passion'.
  (Ruggiero 2015)

There are many examples of how personal observation, frustration, and dissatisfaction, searching for causes, and being sensitive to the implications of situations can yield rich material for writing professional articles. One such example can be found in the notable case of Olga Kanitsaki, AM, formerly professor of transcultural nursing and head of nursing and midwifery at

Royal Melbourne Institute of Technology (RMIT) University in Melbourne (now retired). Kanitsaki first arrived in Australia in the 1960s as a non–English-speaking immigrant from Greece. She later trained and worked as a registered nurse in Melbourne. During the course of her work, Kanitsaki often observed patients of non-English-speaking and culturally diverse backgrounds being treated unfairly and in blatantly prejudicial, soul-destroying, and harmful ways by attending health professionals of the day. When interviewed in 1990 about her experiences, Kanitsaki (1990, p. 16) recounted:

> There was a lot of prejudice. They used to say to me, 'Speak English', when I tried to help an elderly woman or man who couldn't speak English, by translating into Greek. The staff thought I was talking about them. I realised that there were reasons why people I worked with behaved the way they did. In order to understand their insecurities I had to ask how I could help them, rather than becoming defensive or angry about their behaviour.

Recognising the significant implications of cultural diversity for patient safety and quality care and the need for attending health professionals to be educated about these implications, Kanitsaki embarked on a 20-year journey of writing and speaking about cross-cultural issues in healthcare. Her first article entitled 'Acculturation—a new dimension of nursing', published in the *Australian Nurses Journal* in 1983 and based on a clinical case study involving a Greek-born woman facing a leg amputation, is regarded today as a foundation article on the subject of transcultural nursing and healthcare (Kanitsaki, 1983). Of further relevance to this discussion is that Kanitsaki published her article at a time when it was rare and even forbidden by some hospitals for clinical nurses to publish an article in a professional journal. Today, this article continues to be cited by other authors writing on the topic of transcultural healthcare and related issues.

In 1995, Olga Kanitsaki was made a Member in the Order of Australia for her distinguished service to multicultural healthcare and to nursing. In 2000, she was awarded a Doctor of Philosophy degree from Melbourne University and was subsequently appointed as the first professor of transcultural nursing in Australia. Kanitsaki's story is an outstanding example of how personal observations can lead to the writing of influential articles and to the development of an influential and distinguished writing and professional career. When asked in the context of revising this book why she wrote her first article and what motivated her to go on to publish other works during her career, she responded:

> When I first experienced the hospital routines and practices as a student nurse, I was extremely distressed by certain care practices that I witnessed. While these practices were considered normal in 1960s 70s, and 80s, I realised at the time that they were not based on science—rather they were mediated by culture. I was thus very strongly motivated to influence change and improve the experiences and care of patients in hospitals.
>
> I was outspoken at the time but mainly ignored. I remember that, in 1978, I gave my first lecture in a hospital after being invited to speak by another immigrant nurse (who was a tutor at the hospital) to speak about cultural awareness and the changes that needed to be made. This was the beginning of many more speeches I gave in a variety of hospitals and nursing schools at the time.
>
> I desperately wanted to publish my experiences and thoughts regarding the hospital care delivery I had witnessed in regard to immigrant patients of non-English speaking backgrounds. I was aware of the cultural differences

between patients and health professionals and the different expectations each had regarding the delivery of care. I desperately wanted to write about these issues and ensure that the professions were made aware of the difficulties that immigrant patients and their families were facing in hospitals and healthcare settings generally.

I believed that, in addition to me giving speeches about cultural awareness, I needed to publish my observations so that I could influence the health professions generally and specifically nursing. Early in the 1980's, through the Australian Nursing Federation, I was involved in disseminating a new idea imported from America called the 'Nursing Process'. The Nursing Process offered a framework for clinical practice and decision making, but at the time I thought that it was a great framework to use for publishing as well. So, I attempted to write my first article based on my clinical practice and experience as a charge nurse, which I was at the time. I used the framework of the Nursing Process to construct the article. I showed the finalised article to a friend who was an academic. She generously corrected the grammar in the draft article, which I subsequently submitted to the Australian Nursing Journal for consideration. The journal published the article, which was the first of its kind to be published from an Australian perspective on cultural issues in clinical nursing practice. This was my beginning in publishing, which originated from the strong almost painful desire to influence positive change in healthcare delivery by all professionals.

(Kanitsaki, personal communication)

Once you have chosen a topic, there are a number of other considerations that need to be taken into account. Specifically, you need to consider whether:

- you know the subject area well enough to be able write about it
- you feel strongly enough to write about it (for instance, do you have a real passion for the subject area?)
- anyone would seriously disagree with the position or viewpoint you are wishing to advance
- the topic is worth addressing at all.

CHOOSING YOUR AUDIENCE

It is important to be clear right at the outset about *who* is your intended audience. Your intended audience can have an important bearing not only on *what* you write, but also on *how* you write it.

In deciding who your audience is, focused attention must first be given to:

- identifying who, precisely, it is you want to inform (for example, whether your target audience is discipline-specific or multidiscipline in nature, novice or expert, gender-specific or gender-neutral, and so forth)
- deciding what it is you want to inform them about
- clarifying why you want to inform them (what are you trying to achieve by communicating your ideas and views to them)
- choosing the best approach to reach your target audience (e.g., depending on the issue, options include writing a brief report, a case study, a case scenario, correspondence, a critical essay, an opinion article, a policy brief, or a research article)
- choosing the most appropriate publication outlet to reach your target audience (e.g., a specific journal, a book, an anthology, a newsletter, a blog, or a social media platform).

CHOOSING YOUR PUBLICATION OUTLET

In choosing where to get your work published, remember that healthcare professional groups constitute a niche market for commercial publishers. To put this simply, doctors, nurses, midwives, psychologists, occupational therapists, physiotherapists, chiropractors, and the like are recognised as small, specialised groups to whom those in the publishing industry can market journals and books profitably.

Professional niche markets provide aspiring writers (both novice and veteran) with pointed opportunities to publish. By virtue of their specialised knowledge, healthcare professionals not only have a field to write in, but have a ready audience—and market—for whom they can write. In order to exploit this market well, however, prospective writers need to conduct some market research, in other words 'do their homework' to ascertain where the best and most appropriate opportunities lie. In particular, attention needs to be given to ascertaining:

- what is out there already
- who are the relevant editors and who serve on the editorial boards of select journals
- what the editors are looking for
- what journals are appropriate (what kinds of articles do they publish—e.g., do they only publish research reports, or do they accept other types of articles such as critical commentaries, opinion articles, and essays?)
- which publishing companies are appropriate
- what other outlets (e.g., digital media platforms, social media) are appropriate
- the prescribed word limits
- the styles that are used
- what topic to write about and how best to approach it (noting here a key maxim of publishing: 'Think outside the square'

and ask yourself 'Can I approach this topic in a different way to others?').

Once you know what is out there—and what is wanted—it is much easier to pursue your publishing goals. Nevertheless, it is always important to be cautious in making your decision and to choose possible outlets for your work carefully. In making your final decision, consider whether a given outlet:

- will enable you to reach your intended audience
- will give you the scope you need in order to advance the discussion you wish to present—that is, in terms of:
  —specified word limit
  —editorial control
  —aims and objectives of the journal/publishing house
  —timelines
- is reputable (beware of disreputable, unscrupulous, rogue and predatory publishers, and using online sock puppetry accounts; these could all be a disadvantage in the long term to your career or reputation).

PROFESSIONAL JOURNALS

Specialist professional journals constitute the main publishing outlet for healthcare professionals, and when embarking on a writing career, they are the best outlet for your first submission. Before submitting a manuscript to a professional journal for consideration, however, it is important to do two things:

- conduct an analysis of the journals available in your field to make sure you are choosing the most appropriate journal for your work

- ensure that you know and comply with the editorial requirements of the journal to which you have chosen to submit your manuscript.

Conducting an analysis of professional journals

As part of your analysis, you need first to survey the market to ascertain:

- which journals are publishing articles on topics relevant to your field of interest and/or expertise
- what makes each of the journals identified different from each other, for example:
  —who the readers are (if a given journal will reach your intended audience)
  —what information it is seeking
  —what is to be communicated
  —how widely the journal is circulated/distributed
  —what its publication standards are
  —what its Impact Factor is (this can be found in the Journal Citation Reports [JCR] database)
  —whether the journal is indexed on relevant citation indexes, for example, EBSCOHOST, PROQUEST CENTRAL, WEB OF SCIENCE, SCOPUS, MEDLINE CENTRAL, CINAHL (the Cumulative Index to Nursing and Allied Health Literature).
- the implications of submitting work to and having work published in the journal you are considering
- the processes for submitting an article for review and publication in a particular journal
- the editorial requirements of the journal.

Meeting editorial requirements

One of the surest ways of getting a manuscript rejected is to violate the journal's editorial requirements. Several years ago, in the era of surface mail submissions, I had a manuscript rejected outright because of my inadvertent failure to use US English spelling in just *one word*—which, unfortunately, happened to be in the title of the manuscript! (I had spelled the word 'utilised' with an 's' instead of the US English 'utilized'). The manuscript was returned within a few days without being reviewed. All that was attached to the returned manuscript was a photocopied section from what appeared to be the journal's 'Guidelines for Authors' and on which were highlighted in yellow the words emphasising the imperatives of using 'American spelling'. Today, editors are more forgiving and authors whose manuscripts are accepted for publication have the opportunity to correct any stylistic errors before resubmitting their work for publication. Nonetheless, the lesson is clear: always follow stringently the author guidelines of the journal to which you have made a submission.

When preparing a manuscript for submission to a professional journal, it is essential that you obtain, know, and comply with the journal's editorial requirements, which are usually contained in a section headed 'Notes to contributors' or 'Information for authors'. This information usually appears on either the front or back cover of a print journal—or, as is more common today, can be downloaded directly from a publisher's designated website. Some academic publishers also provide 'kits' of comprehensive guidelines and services to authors on how to publish their research and other works (see, for example, the Taylor and Francis 'Author Services' at https://authorservices.taylorandfrancis.com/).

Meeting the editorial requirements of a journal is a matter of common sense, but be aware, particularly, of the following:

1 *Editors*—approach in a professional manner (compose your correspondence carefully).
2 *Manuscript*—comply with the prescribed format (for example, A4 paper, double-spaced, 3 cm margins,

50–100–250-word abstract, key words). Most journals give very specific instructions on how manuscripts should be prepared and submitted.

3 *Timelines*—know and meet timelines (develop a reputation for submitting on or before time). If your manuscript is accepted for publication on the condition that certain amendments are made, ensure that you make the required changes and get the amended manuscript back to the journal within the prescribed timelines. Failure to return an amended manuscript by the prescribed timeline may result in the work not being published. In the case of typeset proofs of an edited manuscript, if these are not returned within the time specified and no reason is given for the delay, they will generally be regarded as having been approved by the author and will be published as edited. If you are having difficulty meeting a deadline, write to the editor and request an extension of time.

4 *Word limit*—write to length (all journals are strict about prescribed word limits and many journals now require word counts to be provided).

5 *Style*—comply with prescribed referencing style; also comply with prescribed spelling requirements. For example, you may be required to use either UK English or US English spelling.

6 *Submission integrity*—manuscripts are generally accepted on the understanding that the content has not been published or submitted elsewhere for publication; most journal guidelines carry a statement to this effect. It is usual practice that once you have submitted your manuscript, you do not submit it elsewhere.

7 *Attribution of authorship*—demonstrate that each of the authors named as either writing or contributing to the manuscript meet the criteria for author attribution as prescribed by the International Committee of Medical Journal

Editors (ICMJE) (the ICMJE criteria will be outlined and discussed in more detail in Chapter 8 of this book).

ACADEMIC BOOK PUBLISHERS

Another (although less accessible) publishing outlet for healthcare professionals is academic book publishing companies. Sometimes the opportunity arises to contribute a chapter to a book being edited by another, or to write a book as a sole author or in collaboration with others.

As in the case of professional journals, before submitting a manuscript to an academic publishing house for consideration, you need to do some preparatory work, notably:

* survey the market for a prospective publisher
* make an initial inquiry through the publisher's website
* formulate a book proposal in keeping with the publisher's guidelines.

As with author guidelines for the submission of journal articles, guidelines on preparing a book proposal and book publishing can also be downloaded directly from a publisher's website.

The academic publishing house Routledge, for example, has a site dedicated to enabling prospective authors to 'find everything you need to know about' the book publishing process (visit www.routledge.com/our-customers/authors/publishing-guidelines).

MARKET SURVEY

As part of your analysis, you need first to survey the market to ascertain:

* which commercial publishers are publishing foundational texts/books on topics relevant to your field of interest and/

or expertise. (This can be undertaken relatively easily by doing an internet search, or a search of your local university library, using the relevant key words pertinent to the subject at issue. Key words which might be helpful in your search can be found by searching the Medical Education Subject Heading [MeSH] index, which can be found by visiting www.ncbi.nlm.nih.gov/mesh/).

- what makes the various book publishers identified different from one another, for example:
  —who the readers are/what market is being targeted
  —what information is being sought
  —who with the company has published a book (what their standing in the field is)
  —how successful texts published by the company are
  —what marketing resources the company has to promote its work
  —what the company's overseas distribution is like
  —what the commercial viability of the company is
  —what the implications of submitting work to and having work published by the book publisher selected are. For instance:
    - what are the restrictions on editorial freedom?
    - what kind of copyright agreement is required?
    - what editing standards will be applied?
    - how do they deal with and relate to authors?
    - what provisions are included in the legal contract?
    - what royalties are paid? (these can range from 3–15% for academic texts, although author advocacy groups recommend that royalties should not be less than 10%)
    - what are the processes for submitting a book proposal for consideration?

WRITING A BOOK

It is not far-fetched to have a dream of writing a book one day. Moreover, as stated earlier, most academic publishing houses will accept an inquiry about a book proposal. There are, however, several steps that need to be followed.

Initial inquiry

The first step is to make an inquiry. The objective of forwarding an initial inquiry about a proposed book idea is to generate interest in your work and to convince an acquisition editor that your proposal is a viable proposition. The general process you should follow in your approaches is:

- make sure you are approaching the publishing company in the manner as advised on their website
- obtain a copy of the company's guidelines for submitting a book proposal
- write all correspondence concerning your proposal in a professional manner and include a trustworthy email address for a reply
- keep a record of the companies that you submit proposals to (i.e., to whom you sent the manuscript and when).

Formulating a book proposal

As noted earlier in this chapter, publishing companies have dedicated guidelines and related resources that are readily available for prospective authors on how to structure and formulate a book proposal. Typically, publishers require:

1 *Information about the author*
   - Name, qualifications, and professional affiliations
   - Contact details: email, postal address, telephone, and—in some instances—fax numbers (business and private)

- A brief description of your rationale for writing the book and your qualifications for doing so (if you have a successful record of publishing in professional journals, this will enhance your credentials for writing a book).

2 *Information about the proposed book*
- A complete book outline, including is stated aims, and a brief synopsis of the content of each chapter
- The anticipated length of the manuscript and the proposed work plan and completion date
- Three representative sample chapters
- The primary (and secondary) market and the approximate numbers involved (e.g., how many readers, its teaching features)
- The specific advantages your book will have over other competing works (including its 'sell points', professional suitability, and institutional support)
- Reports on your other work.

In addition, publishers may require prospective authors to complete an 'Author marketing questionnaire' which they provide.

NEWSLETTERS, NEWSPAPERS, BLOGS, AND SOCIAL MEDIA PLATFORMS

Another outlet for publishing a work is a profession's or an organisation's newsletter, or independent online newspapers (e.g., *The Conversation* and campus newspapers such as *Campus Review*). Social media platforms such as Twitter or Instagram also provide important opportunities to publish, noting that both of these platforms have high levels of engagement by healthcare professionals and are increasingly recognised as providing scholars with 'a significant platform for engaging in and disseminating scholarship' (Acquaviva et al., 2020, p. 3).

Being less formal in tone and format than peer-reviewed journals and texts, wonderful opportunities for aspiring writers to see their work 'in print' can be provided by newsletters, newspapers, blogs, and social media platforms. Furthermore, editors of newsletters are *always* on the lookout for material and often actively solicit contributions from associates in order to keep the publication viable.

Although contributions to newsletters and other print or social media are typically—and by necessity—smaller than those generally published in journals and texts, they nevertheless require the same degree of focus, discipline, and 'good writing' as their counterparts (*The Conversation*, for example, requires a high standard of writing and integrity from its contributing authors—see https://theconversation.com/au). In several respects, they require *more* discipline on account of authors having to express their views in a concise number of words (in some cases, fewer than 500 words). Making an impact on readers in just 500 words is a challenge—even for veteran authors. This is sometimes referred to as 'The government minister in the lift' test: if, by chance, you found yourself in the lift (called an 'elevator' in some countries) with the health minister of your government, how would you use this opportunity—What issue would you raise? How would you approach it? If you just happened to have a copy of a small 500-word commentary in your pocket, would you share it with and invite the minister to read it? Would the opening line in your commentary 'hook' the minister into listening to you and reading the entire text?

The key to writing a successful contribution for a newsletter, blog, or social media platforms is to write on a topic that is interesting and provides information that is useful to the stakeholders. In order to pitch your contribution at the right level, it is important that you clarify:

- who is producing the newsletter/newspaper/blog/social media platform, and for what purpose
- the aims and objectives of the newsletter/newspaper/blog/social media platform
- who the readers are
- what they are reading for (that is, what are their interests, information needs, and areas of concern?)
- how widely the newsletter/newspaper/blog/social media platform is circulated/distributed
- the circumstances under which constituents are likely to be reading the newsletter/newspaper/blog/social media platform (will these outlets engage a wide audience?)
- what, if any, implications there might be (good and bad) of you writing for the newsletter/newspaper/blog/social media platform
- what the timelines for production are.

CONCLUSION

Getting started on a new work can be an intimidating experience, even for the most experienced of writers. In order to overcome this 'block', it is important that you are clear about your writing goals and focus consistently and persistently on achieving them. Be very discerning in choosing a topic, deciding your audience, and selecting your publishing outlet. You should also find a mentor—someone who can be a 'friendly critic' and who can support you on your writing journey. Once you have decided these things and have in place the necessary supports, you are then in a position to engage fully in the process of writing (the subject of Chapter 3). This is where the real work begins.

EXERCISES

1 Complete the following statements:
   - My mission as a writer is to: ....
   - My reasons for wanting to write are: ....
   - What I most wish to achieve with my writing is:
     ....

2 Compare your mission statement, reasons for wanting to write, and your stated writing aspirations with the statements of another aspiring writer and discuss the similarities and differences in your responses.

3 Drawing on your own personal observations and experience, identify a topic on which you would like to write an article or commentary.

4 Evaluate how strongly you feel about the topic you have chosen, whether you know the subject area well enough to write about it, and whether the topic is worth writing about at all (if this evaluation yields a poor result, choose another topic).

5 Decide what approach is best suited to addressing the topic or issue you have chosen to write about—e.g., a brief report, a case study, a case scenario, correspondence, a critical essay, an opinion article, a policy brief, or a research article.

6 Survey a list of professional journals in your field and compare what each has to offer. Identify two or three journals in which you would like to have an article published. Set a realistic timeframe for submitting articles to these journals for review and publication.

7 Find a mentor who is willing to support you in achieving your publishing goals.

REFERENCES

Acquaviva, K. D., Mugele, J., Abadilla, N., Adamson, T., Bernstein, S. L., Bhayani, R. K., . . . & Trudell, A. M. (2020). Documenting social media engagement as scholarship: A new model for assessing academic accomplishment for the health professions. *Journal of Medical Internet Research, 22*(12), e25070. DOI: 10.2196/25070

Blythe, W. (Ed.). (1998). *Why I write: Thoughts on the craft of fiction.* Little, Brown and Company.

Bryant, R. (1999). *Anybody can write: A playful approach: Ideas for the aspiring writer, the beginner, the blocked writer.* New World Library.

Edelstein, S. (1999). *100 things every writer needs to know, perigee.* The Berkley Publishing Group.

hooks, b. (1999). *Remembered rapture: The writer at work.* Henry Holt and Company.

Kanitsaki, O. (1983). Acculturation–A new dimension in nursing. *The Australian Nurses' journal. Royal Australian Nursing Federation, 12*(5), 42–5.

Kanitsaki, O. (1990). Dignifying difference: Multicultural health care. In *Interview by P. Romios in the healthsharing reader: Women speak about health.* Healthsharing Women, Pandora.

King, S. (2000). *On writing: A memoir.* Hodder & Stoughton.

Rowling, J. K. (2019). *On writing.* Retrieved from www.jkrowling.com/opinions/on-writing/

Ruggiero, V. (2015). *The art of thinking: A guide to critical and creative thought* (11th ed.). Pearson.

3 | THE WRITING PROCESS

INTRODUCTION

The process of writing begins the moment you decide to write *and* physically sit down to commence the work. Thereafter, as Stephen King (2000, p. 122) notes, the work 'is always accomplished one word at a time'. Meanwhile, the challenge once you start writing is not merely to keep focused on what you are doing and to keep writing until the work has been completed, but to write *well*.

Most books addressing the art, craft, and science of successful writing acknowledge that an essential ingredient of 'good' writing is *style*. As the veteran writer Majorie Holmes (1969, p. 107) points out in her classic text *Writing the Creative Article*:

> Style is important. Of style, Aristotle said, 'it is not enough to know what to say; we must also say it in the right way.' The first impression an editor gets from any piece of writing is the author's style. The subject may be a good one, the words sufficient—like clothes, they may *cover* it; but if they are sloppy, prosaic or dull, or merely inappropriate, the editor has to drive himself [sic] to get through the manuscript.

The question is: what is style, and can it be taught?

THE ELEMENTS OF STYLE

At its most basic, style is 'the effective use of words to engage the human mind' (Pinker, 2014, p. 2). In regard to an author's particular style this may be described as '*your* way of writing'— the expression of your personality as an author (Holmes, 1969,

DOI: 10.4324/9781003413226-3

p. 108) (Emphasis Original). A more substantive definition of style is:

> The art of clear, effective, and readable writing. The rhythm that makes a sentence sound right to the mental ear. The ruthless cutting out of phrases that only clutter and impede this special music. And always, always, the patient, painstaking search for the perfect combination of words and phrases that will create this mental music and express what is to be said in the most moving and effective way.
>
> (Holmes, 1969, p. 107)

WRITING WITH 'VOICE'

Style can also be defined as writing that expresses or carries the author's 'voice', without which the writing might be 'dead'. Peter Elbow's (1998, pp. 287–288) views on this issue are worth quoting at length. He writes:

> Writing with no voice is dead, mechanical, faceless. It lacks any sound. Writing with no voice may be saying something true, important, or new; it may be logically organized; it may even be a work of genius. But it is as though the words came through some kind of mixer rather than uttered by a person. Extreme lack of voice is characteristic of bureaucratic memos, technical engineering writing, much sociology, many textbooks . . . . Nobody is home here. In its extreme form, no voice is the army-manual of style. But the sad truth is that the careful writing of most people lacks voice . . . .
>
> Voice, in contrast, is what most people have in their speech but lack in their writing—namely, a sound or texture—the sound of 'them'. We recognize most of our friends on the phone before they say who they are. A few people get their voice into their writing. When you read a

letter or something else they've written, it has the sound of them. It feels as though writing with voice has life in it.

Sometimes a writer's style may be so strong that others can recognise it without knowing the identity of the author. For example, I was once informed by a publisher: 'Your manuscript reviewed very well. You might also like to know that one of the reviewers responded, "I don't know who wrote this chapter, but I bet it was Megan-Jane Johnstone—it *sounds* like her" '.

CAN STYLE BE TAUGHT?

Many ask whether style can be taught. The short answer to this question is: yes, no, maybe. In at least one fundamental sense, style is elusive in much the same way that 'rhythm or good taste or passion' is elusive, and hence not something that can be taught (Holmes, 1969, p. 107). In another sense, style can be 'taught' in that writers can be shown how to *develop* and *improve* their style. According to Holmes (1969, p. 108), there are two cardinal rules for improving and developing style:

- by writing—not just occasionally, but regularly
- by developing an awareness of the style of others—notably by reading and studying the work of others.

On this latter point, William Zinsser (2019, p. 30) advises:

> Make a habit of reading what is written today and what has been written by earlier masters. Writing is learned by imitation. If anyone asked me how I learned to write, I'd say I learned by reading men and women who were doing the kind of writing I wanted to do and trying to figure out how they did it. But cultivate the best models.

Holmes advocates the following specific strategies for developing your own writing style:

- expose yourself to the kinds of things you want to write about
- read widely (not just one author)
- mark passages that please you and reread them, noting why they please you
- underscore the good figures of speech—count their frequency and taste their flavour
- read the works just before you sit down to write

  (adapted from Holmes, 1969, pp. 109–10).

THE PRINCIPLES OF STYLE

The development of a good writing style—like the development of good conduct—can be guided by a set of principles. Some such principles, or 'secrets of style' as Marjorie Holmes refers to them, are:

1. aim for simplicity
2. avoid trite phrases and clichés
3. use figures of speech appropriately
4. avoid euphemisms, slang and colloquialisms
5. choose your words carefully (seek the 'right' word; avoid rare and difficult words)
6. avoid repeating key words (unless for emphasis or effect)
7. avoid redundancy
8. use alliteration
9. keep sentences as short as possible
10. develop a feel for rhythm
11. be original.

(adapted from Holmes, 1969, pp. 110–22)

Another crucial characteristic of style is what award-winning US cognitive scientist and public intellectual Steven Pinker (2014, p. 139) calls the 'arcs of coherence'—which, he contends, are essential to ensure that readers 'grasp the topic, get the point, keep track of the players, and see how one idea follows from another'. Clarifying what he means by the notion of 'arcs of coherence', Pinker (2014, p. 186) explains:

> a coherent text is a designed object: an ordered tree of sections within sections, crisscrossed by arcs that track topics, points, actors, and themes, and held together by connectors that tie one proposition to the next. Like other objects, it comes about not by accident but by drafting a blueprint, attending to details, and maintaining a sense of harmony and balance.

Aim for simplicity

The key to good writing is *simplicity*—that is, saying what you mean in a clear, direct, and simple (though engaging) manner. To achieve simplicity in your work, follow these steps:

1 write the work
2 take a 'cooling-off' period
3 return to the work after a few days (or, if time is of the essence, at the very least after a night's sleep)
4 reread it
5 search for anything that detracts from what you mean to say or obscures its clarity
6 remove any words, views, or expressions that are superfluous.

(Holmes, 1969; Zinsser, 2019)

Many writers think that using 'big words' (for example, 'accede to' versus 'allow'; 'acquiesce' versus 'agree'; 'reside' versus 'live') and discipline-exclusive jargon enhances the merits and profundity of what they are writing (for a comparative list of common *complex* versus *simple* words, see Manser & Curtis, 2002, pp. 205–207). In reality, however, jargon and big words often obscure what the writer is trying to say and may make their work largely inaccessible and meaningless to others. Sometimes, of course, it is genuinely difficult to avoid discipline-specific jargon. For instance, in my writing on ethics and bioethics, words like 'ethics', 'morality', 'rights', 'duties', 'deontology', 'teleology', and so forth, are often critical to the discussion I am advancing and, on account of having specific philosophic meanings, not able to be avoided. To overcome the problem of these words possibly making my writing obscure and unclear—especially when writing for a novice audience—I explain up front what these terms mean.

The hallmark of a 'good' writer is someone who can make complex ideas accessible and meaningful. Furthermore, as Holmes (1969, p. 111) correctly argues, 'A good mind with a good idea should strive to make that idea understood'. Obscurity, suggests Holmes, is *not* the mark of profundity and should be avoided at all costs.

One process that can be used to keep a check on the use of words whose meanings may be obscure to others is to:

- identify the 'big words' in your work
- ask yourself whether the inclusion of these word is really necessary, or whether there are other simpler words that could be used (to assist in the search for simpler words, consult a dictionary and/or a thesaurus)
- seek the advice of an 'ally reader' on whether the sections of writing you are concerned about are as obscure as you think (beware also of being overly self-critical).

Avoid trite phrases and clichés

Clichés in writing are regarded as being the 'kiss of death' to a manuscript—not least because they undermine the process of continuing originality that is so critical to achieving stylish writing (Zinsser, 2019, p. 165). On this, Pinker (2014, p. 46) offers the following frank advice: 'Avoid clichés like the plague'.

According to William Zinsser (2019, p. 165) if you want to give your readers a taste of something fresh, use words and expressions that have 'surprise, strength and precision'. Words that do not have these qualities should not be used. The following are some examples of clichés:

- 'At the end of the day'
- 'At the cutting edge'
- 'The bottom line is . . . '
- 'While there's life, there's hope'
- 'When push comes to shove . . . '
- 'It was too good to be true'
- 'To explore every avenue'
- 'The powers that be'
- 'The eye-watering/eye-popping costs of . . . '
- 'You don't have to be a rocket scientist to figure out . . . '
- 'Few and far between'.

It is generally accepted by those writing about writing that clichés should be avoided unless you are an extremely experienced writer with the capacity to use a cliché in a deliberate, clever, and surprising way to emphasise a point. One way of achieving this is by treating the phrase 'contrapuntally'—that is, by turning it about. The technique of 'contrapuntal turnabout' is discussed later in this chapter.

Use figures of speech appropriately

A *figure of speech* is 'an expression of language, such as a simile, metaphor, or personification, by which the usual or literal meaning of the word is not employed' (*Collins English Dictionary*, 2014).

The decision to use figures of speech in written work needs to be considered carefully. Like clichés, if they are not used skilfully, they can be detrimental to a manuscript. *Mixing* figures of speech can be especially problematic since this can confuse both the image and associated point that the writer is trying to make. On this latter point, Holmes cautions, 'Better no images at all than mixed ones' (1969, p. 115).

Having said this, using figures of speech skilfully can be a very useful device to:

- emphasise a point
- add life, rhetorical force, and interest to your style
- generally enhance the coherency and integrity of your work.

A good example of how a figure of speech can be used successfully to emphasise a point—and to do so succinctly and with power—can be found by looking at Dr Bob Brown, a former Australian politician and leading figure in the Australian conservation movement. One of Dr Brown's great talents is his ability to use metaphors effectively and to create pictures with words in order to both explain and emphasise a point. One example of this is his reported comment that, 'Flooding the Franklin [a wilderness area situated in the State of Tasmania] would be like putting a scratch across the *Mona Lisa* or across a Beethoven record'.

Commenting on Bob Brown's capacity to use picturesque speech, Jonathan West writes:

When someone says, 'we're just putting a little road through a wilderness area,' he [Bob Brown] is able to create a picture by saying 'that's like putting a scratch across the face of the *Mona Lisa*. The vast majority of the *Mona Lisa* is intact, but the scratch spoils it.' The long, detailed, technical explanation about the way in which the road would reduce the amount of wilderness square kilometres would have nothing like the same impact as a simple word image like that.

(West, quoted in Thompson, 2000, pp. 51–52)

Avoid euphemisms, slang, and colloquialisms

A euphemism (from the Greek *euphēmismos*, meaning 'sounding good') is an inoffensive word or phrase that is substituted for a word or phrase that may be considered offensive, embarrassing, taboo, or hurtful. Examples include: 'passed away' (instead of died), 'ethnic cleansing' (instead of genocide), and 'passed wind' (instead of farted).

The use of euphemisms in formal writing is not generally encouraged since it can be misleading and inappropriate. One reason for this is that origin may be obscure and, since euphemisms cannot be interpreted literally, they can be misunderstood—especially if the audience does not share a common understanding of their meaning (Yamasaki, 2022). Another reason relates to the use of euphemisms creating a casual tone of the writing, which may have the undesirable effect of undermining the seriousness of the subject matter being considered. This does not mean that euphemisms should never be used. Rather, if they are used, they need to be used in a masterly way. George Orwell (1984), for example, used euphemisms in a masterly way in his celebrated dystopian novel *Nineteen Eighty-Four*, first published in 1949. As Yamasaki (2022) notes, the euphemisms used in this novel obscured the dangerous subjects that each of the political authorities featured in the novel were responsible for—e.g., 'the Party' (a euphemism for the government), the 'Ministry of Truth' (a euphemism for the ministry in charge of propaganda), and the 'Ministry of Peace' (a euphemism for the ministry in charge of war).

Slang refers to vocabulary (characteristically metaphorical in nature) that falls outside of the standard form of language; a colloquialism is similar to slang in that it refers to an informal expression that is appropriate only in certain contexts and conversations. Examples include:

- 'Buckley's chance' (Australian and New Zealand slang for 'no chance at all')
- 'cocky' (Australian informal for 'cockatoo', a native bird, or New Zealand and Australian slang for 'a cow farmer'; also US and Canadian slang for 'someone who is overly sure of themselves')
- 'dilly' (US and Canadian slang for 'a person or thing that is remarkable'; in Australia and New Zealand it slang for quite the opposite and refers to 'someone who is remarkably silly')
- 'wally' (general slang for 'stupid person').

Like euphemisms, slang and colloquialisms can be misunderstood, can confuse readers, and can generally undermine the quality of formal writing—and for these reasons, they are best avoided.

Choose your words carefully

Good writing is both an art and craft. It fundamentally involves the art of carefully crafting words into expressions that have the capacity to convey images and ideas with strength, precision, and originality. Good writing makes an impression on the minds of its readers; depending on the subject matter, good writing also has the capacity to change lives.

A critical ingredient of good writing is the careful selection of words and crafting them into each line of writing. No effort should be spared in searching for and selecting the 'right' words and, once found, using them with discipline and care. As Conroy (1998, p. 57) reflects:

> I try to write down every word with caution and a sense of craft, as though I were carving hieroglyphics on the tomb of a well-loved king. Writing is both hard labor and one of the most pleasant forms that fanaticism can take. I take infinite care in how a sentence sounds to me.

As already mentioned, the use of 'big words' and rare or difficult words is not good writing; moreover, the use of such words is likely to confound readers and to cause them to feel frustrated and irritated. Frustrating the reader is not a good outcome; among other things, it can lead to a 'lost reader'— and ultimately, a lost audience.

Choosing the right word means you need to know the correct meanings of the words you are using. This may seem obvious, but it is surprising how often writers overlook this crucial point. Often, we think we know the meaning of a given word, only to discover at some later point (either in conversation with others or when consulting a dictionary) that it may in fact have quite a different meaning to what we thought.

It is important to be mindful that language is not static and that the meaning of words can and do change over time. Evidence of this can be found in the 20-volume *Oxford English Dictionary* where discussion on the definition of a word, its origins, and its different meanings can run into *pages*, not merely paragraphs.

Since words are the essential ingredients of writing, it is essential that all writers get into the habit of using dictionaries. I would add that all writers should also get into the habit of using *different* dictionaries—e.g., the *Oxford English Dictionary*, the *Collins English Dictionary*, and *Webster's Dictionary*.

Reasons for this are that each of these dictionaries may offer a slightly different perspective on the meaning of a given word, which can be thought-provoking and add substance to a discussion being advanced.

Using the wrong words—or using words that are inappropriate—may prove to be not only embarrassing for a writer but, more seriously, may undermine the meaning, purpose, significance, and integrity of a writer's work. One way to avoid this situation is to care deeply about your writing and about the words that you ultimately choose to use. On this point, Holmes (1969, p. 119) advises:

> The truly creative writer cares deeply about words—enough to take infinite pains to make his [or her] writing style as nearly perfect as possible. This means a constant quest to find the one word that most precisely expresses his [or her] thought . . . . Good writing can only come from this quality of deep caring, and this willingness to work toward perfection. Bad writing comes sometimes less from lack of talent than from sheer carelessness.

Avoid repeating key words

It is easy, when writing, to fall into the trap of repeating key words. All writers do it—most unintentionally, some even carelessly—but either way, rarely are they used with good effect. Unless there is an intended purpose behind repeating key words, such as to emphasise or underscore a crucial point, this practice is best avoided. Holmes (1969, p. 118) crafted the following paragraph as an example of tardy repetitious writing:

> I cannot tell you how moved I am to come here and try to dedicate this ground. As I move toward this ground and tried to think how to dedicate it I realised that I had dedicated myself

to a task which cannot be done. This ground was already dedicated, I thought, by the death of the men who died.

Although it is best to avoid repeating key words, this does not mean that there is no place for utilising the technique of 'repetition' as a creative device in writing.

Some writers are able to skilfully use the technique of repeating key words with good effect. A famous example of this can be found in Martin Luther King's legendary 'I Have a Dream' speech, delivered on the steps at the Lincoln Memorial in Washington, DC on 28 August 1963 (an archival pdf copy of this speech can be downloaded from www.archives.gov/files/social-media/transcripts/transcript-march-pt3-of-3-2602934.pdf). In this speech Dr King repeated the words 'I have a dream' eight times, and the words 'Let freedom ring' seven times in his concluding comments.

There are other poignant repetitions in King's speech, which work to great effect. For instance, when referring to the level of dissatisfaction among Black Americans concerning their lack of civil rights, King (1963, emphasis added) wrote:

> *We can never be satisfied* as long as our bodies, heavy with the fatigue of travel, cannot gain lodging in the motels of the highways and the hotels of the cities. *We cannot be satisfied as* long as the Negro's basic mobility is from a smaller ghetto to a larger one. *We can never be satisfied* as long as a Negro in Mississippi cannot vote and a Negro in New York believes he has nothing for which to vote. No, no, *we are not satisfied*, and *we will not be satisfied* until justice rolls down like waters and righteousness like a mighty stream.

In anticipation of Black Americans eventually succeeding in achieving the civil rights and freedom they sought, and how this would be heralded, King concluded his speech by quoting the words from an old Negro spiritual, ' "Free at last! Free at last! Thank God Almighty, we are free at last!" ' (Incidentally, King's speech is also full of rich examples of the effective use of figures of speech; one example is, 'Let us not seek to satisfy our thirst for freedom by drinking from the cup of bitterness and hatred'.)

The words used in King's speech demonstrate that repetition can be used intentionally, powerfully, and with good effect. The key is to be *careful* in the way you use these. As Holmes (1969, p. 122) points out, it is the 'careless, unnecessary repetitions that clutter your style and that editors deplore'.

In order to avoid careless repetitions in your work:

- take care in the original crafting of the work
- take a 'cooling off' period
- re-read the work (or have a mentor or friendly critic read the work) and search actively for any repetitions
- remove repeated words that serve no purpose and/or have no effect in terms of emphasising a point.

Avoid redundancy

In language, words or expressions are generally considered to be redundant when they are *tautological*—that is, they 'merely repeat elements of the meaning already conveyed' (*Collins English Dictionary*, 2014). Expressions can also be redundant when they are verbose—that is, when they contain an excess of words that focus on insignificant detail.

Some notable examples of redundancy include:

- *yellow jaundice*
- *sugar diabetes*
- *two twins*
- 'will the funds available be *adequate enough*' (versus, 'will the funds available be adequate')

- 'the older residents could now climb the stairs *safely and not get hurt*' (versus 'the older residents could now climb the stairs safely')
- '*apparently* the Chief Executive resigned *ostensibly* for health reasons' (versus, 'apparently the Chief Executive resigned for health reasons' or 'the Chief Executive resigned ostensibly for health reasons').

Tips for avoiding redundancy in your work include:

- when writing, do not labour a point unnecessarily
- take a 'cooling-off' period
- reread the work for redundancies
- remove any redundancies.

Use alliteration

Alliteration, defined as 'the occurrence of the same letter or sound at the beginning of adjacent or closely connected words' (*Oxford English Dictionary*, 2023), is another technique that can be used to add life, rhythm, and uniqueness to a writer's style. More commonly associated with poetry and tongue twisters (for example, 'Peter Piper picked a peck of pickled peppers'), many writers overlook this device as a stylish writing technique. Like other creative writing techniques, however, it needs to be applied with craft and skill if it is to work effectively.

Alliteration can be used powerfully and effectively in titles of works, in an opening or a concluding paragraph, and in the general body of a work. For example:

Titles—*The Sense of Style* (Pinker, 2014), *Moral Minds* (Hauser, 2006), *Burning Books* (Fishburn, 2008), *Cruel Compassion: Psychiatric Control of Society's Unwanted* (Szasz, 1994).
Opening paragraph—'Five score years ago, a great American, in whose symbolic shadow we stand signed the Emancipation

Proclamation' (King, 1963, opening sentence to his 'I Have a Dream' speech). Note how the 's' sounds add smoothness and rhythm to his opening statement.

General body—'Just as a sto*pp*ed clock can bear *p*ermanent witness to the exact time of a *p*articular atrocity, so the memory of a *p*articular event in our *p*ast can have the *p*ower to close off the future and sto*p* our life' (Holloway, 2002, p. 32).

Keep sentences as short as possible

Another critical feature of a good writing style is *readability*. Readability of a work can be enhanced greatly by keeping sentences short and to the point. Some sentences will, of course, need to be longer than others, depending on what is being expressed. Nevertheless, there is *always* room for improvement.

When I first started writing as a university undergraduate student in the early 1980s, I wrote long, convoluted sentences in my assignments. Aware that I had a problem (one day I barely passed an assignment when I had expected to get a higher grade), I approached a very patient study-skills teacher for assistance. On my first visit, the teacher gently pointed out to me that one of the sentences in this assignment (I had given it to her for feedback) contained more than 60 words and that several other sentences contained only slightly fewer words than that. I learned valuable lessons that day:

- all sentences in a work need to be examined carefully
- long sentences can always be improved, either by being 'broken' into smaller sentences or by having unnecessary words and phrases deleted
- never underestimate the value of a mentor or friendly reader who is willing to critique your work and who can be trusted to pick you up on your blind spot when it comes to writing long sentences.

Develop a feel for rhythm

Rhythm, the periodic or regular recurrence of sound or movement, is perhaps more commonly associated with music than with writing. Yet rhythm is just as important to good writing as it to good music. Furthermore, as William Zinsser (2019, p. 31) advises, 'considerations of sound and rhythm should be woven through everything you write'.

The best way to get a sense of the rhythm (or lack of rhythm) in your own writing is to read it aloud to yourself. By reading your work aloud, you can 'both hear and feel' its rhythm through speech.

Zinsser (2019, p. 32) states that he writes 'entirely by ear and read[s] everything aloud before letting [his work] go out into the world'. I also read my writing aloud to myself. I listen for its rhythm, and note where it is lacking. When reading aloud, I note where there exists a clutter of words, and where there is a need for pause and punctuation. Over the years, many students have told me that I 'speak like I write'. The reality is that I write like I speak.

There are many ways to cultivate rhythm in your writing. One way is to study the rhythm in the writing of others. A good place to start would be to read the speeches written by Martin Luther King (these can be accessed via the American Writers' Museum at https://americanwritersmuseum.org/martin-luther-king-jr-quotes-and-speeches/).

Many of the world's greatest speeches have been archived and can be downloaded freely from the internet (see, for example, *35 Greatest Speeches in History*, online at www.artofmanliness.com/character/knowledge-of-men/the-35-greatest-speeches-in-history/). Audible versions of great speeches can also be accessed, such as Audible's *The Greatest Speeches of All Time* (www.audible.com.au/pd/The-Greatest-Speeches-of-All-Time-Audiobook/B00FO8AF30).

Other useful resources include:

- *Lend Me Your Ears: Great Speeches in History* (Introduction by William Safire, 1997)
- *Speeches That Changed the World: The Stories and Transcripts of the Moments that Made History* (Introduction by Simon Sebag Montefiore, 2005)
- *50 Speeches That Made the Modern World: Famous Speeches from Women's Rights to Human Rights* (Edited by Burnet, 2016).

Be original

Originality—the ability to create something fresh, new, and unusual—is another important ingredient of style. And, like style, it rests just as much on skill, focus, and hard work as it does on talent, intuition, and creative imagination. While the work of some writers is clearly more original than the work of others, there are nevertheless ways in which originality in style can be enhanced and improved. For example, you can draw on the techniques of:

- 'lateral thinking' and 'thinking outside the square' advocated by the tactician and provocateur Edward de Bono (for a succinct summary of de Bono's many works, see Dudgeon, 2001)
- creative and critical thinking advocated by Ruggiero (2015), a pioneer and author in the field of critical and creative thinking.

Using the contrapuntal device (described in the following sub-section) can also enhance originality as can using the various other style techniques already discussed in this chapter. Being passionately and almost fanatically interested in what you are writing is another means of enhancing originality. As Zinsser (2019, p. 172) concludes:

> Living is the trick. Writers who write interestingly tend to be men and women who keep themselves interested. That's almost the whole point of becoming a writer.

The contrapuntal device

A little-known technique for enhancing writing style is the contrapuntal device—a counterpoint technique whereby a phrase, such as a cliché or figure of speech, is 'turned about'. This technique, also referred to tautologically as the *contrapuntal turnabout*, can give a work what William Safire (1997, p. 19) calls 'quotable nuggets'.

There are many famous examples of contrapuntal expressions. For example, Abraham Lincoln used the device to switch 'the cynical "might is right" to the moral "right makes might"' (Safire, 1997, p. 19). Similarly, John F. Kennedy used the device to switch the pessimistic 'never negotiate out of fear' to the optimistic 'never fear to negotiate' (Safire, 1997, p. 19). Other examples are:

- 'Not everything that counts can be counted, and not everything that can be counted counts' (commonly although incorrectly attributed to Albert Einstein—https://quoteinvestigator. com/2010/05/26/everything-counts-einstein/).
- 'The second, and more reliable, method [for achieving inner contentment] is not to have what we want but rather to want and appreciate what we have' (His Holiness the Dalai Lama & Cutler, 1998, p. 29).
- 'We cannot live within the past, but the past lives within us' (the late Charlie Perkins, Aboriginal leader and activist, dedication and postscript to the film *One Night the Moon* which was directed by Rachel Perkins, his daughter and a noted Australian filmmaker).

Drafting and redrafting

A key part of writing is the process of *drafting* and *redrafting* the work. All writing initially is a draft—a *preliminary* work—since rarely, if at all, is a work word perfect from the outset and almost always will it require at least some amendment. Some works, of course, will require more or less drafting and redrafting than others, depending on the nature of the work and experience of the author, but ultimately, no writing process is complete until the drafting/redrafting process is complete.

Many writers (especially novice writers) baulk at the prospect and experience of having to redraft their work (students writing theses get particularly discouraged by this process). Some writers, however, rightly embrace the redrafting phase as a kind of 'quality control' of their writing (Dunn, 1999, p. 89) and as an opportunity to craft an exemplary piece of work—an attitude that often brings rich rewards. For example, the Russian novelist, short story writer and philosopher Leo Tolstoy (1828–1910), author of the two monumental novels *War and Peace* and *Anna Karenina*, is reputed to have gone through and rewritten his first novel *War and Peace* eight times and was still making corrections on the final galley proofs of the work (Carver, 1983, p. 209). Both of these works became classics and remain in print.

Redrafting a work is just as critical as the original drafting of the work. Your work's success may ultimately depend on this process, provided it is done well. One reason for this is that it enables you to check that the principles of style have been upheld and to make amendments if they have not been. Redrafting provides you with an opportunity to check that:

- the work has been written in a clear, direct, and simple manner
- trite phrases and clichés have been avoided
- figures of speech have been used appropriately
- the right words have been chosen, and rare and difficult words avoided

- repetitions have been avoided or, if used, handled in a skilful and effective manner
- redundancies have been avoided
- alliteration has been used appropriately
- sentences are of an appropriate length, and are shortened if too long
- the work is read aloud and checked for rhythm
- the final work demonstrates the hallmarks of originality
- the work has come together as a coherent, accessible, and meaningful whole.

CONCLUSION

To produce 'good writing', it is essential to apply the elements and principles of style. The key element of style is writing with personality and voice. Through regular practice, mentoring, and exposure to the unique styles of other writers, a writing style can be developed and improved. A good writing style, in turn, can be developed and improved by upholding the principles of style that have as their ultimate purpose the production of writing that is readable, meaningful, original, memorable, and successful. These principles also underscore the point that it is only by sitting down and writing—and, at the appropriate time, rewriting a work—that the job of writing gets done.

EXERCISES

1 Make a list of authors whose writing styles you admire.
2 Study these authors' works and note the 'secrets' of their style.

3 Examine your own work (for example, an essay written for a university course, a journal article you may have had published) and note the extent to which you have upheld (or not upheld) the principles of style and where improvements could be made.

4 Note the use of alliteration in the discussion advanced in the remaining chapters of this book.

REFERENCES

Burnet, A. (Ed.). (2016). *50 speeches that made the modern world: Famous speeches from women's rights to human rights*. Chambers.

Carver, R. (1983). The art of fiction No. 76. *The Paris Review, 88*, 193–221.

Collins English Dictionary. (2014). Figure of speech. In *Collins English dictionary* (12th ed.). HarperCollins Publishers.

Conroy, P. (1998). Stories. In W. Blythe (Ed.), *Why I write: Thoughts on the craft of fiction* (pp. 47–60). Little, Brown and Company.

Dudgeon, P. (2001). *Breaking out of the box: The biography of Edward De Bono*. Hodder Headline.

Dunn, I. (1999). *The Writer's Guide: A companion to writing for pleasure or publication*. Allen & Unwin, Sydney.

Elbow, P. (1998). *Writing with power: Techniques for mastering the writing process* (2nd ed.). Oxford University Press.

Fishburn, M. (2008). *Burning books*. Palgrave MacMillan.

Fishman, R. (2000). *Creative wisdom for writers*. Allen & Unwin.

Hauser, M. D. (2006). *Moral minds: the nature of right and wrong*. Harper Perennial.

His Holiness the Dalai Lama and Cutler, H. (1998). *The art of happiness: A handbook for living*. Hodder.

Holloway, R. (2022). *On forgiveness: How can we forgive the unforgivable?* Canongate Books.

Holmes, M. (1969). *Writing the creative article*. The Writer, Inc.

King, M. L. (1963). *I have a dream*. Retrieved from http://web66. coled.umn.edu/new/MLK/MLK.html

King, S. (2000). *On writing: A memoir*. Hodder & Stoughton.

Manser, M., & Curtis, S. (2002). *The penguin writer's manual*. Penguin Books.

Montefiore, S. S. (2005) *Speeches that changed the world: The stories and transcripts of the moments that made history*. Murdoch Books.

Orwell, G. (1984). *Nineteen eighty-four*. Penguin Modern Classics.

Oxford English Dictionary (OED). (2023). Alliteration, n. In *OED online*. Oxford University Press.

Pinker, S. (2014). *The sense of style: The thinking person's guide to writing in the 21st century*. Penguin Random House.

Ruggiero, V. (2015). *The art of thinking: A guide to critical and creative thought* (11th ed.). Pearson.

Safire, W. (1997). *Lend me your ears: Great speeches in history, revised and expanded edition*. W.W. Norton & Company.

Szasz, T. (1994). *Cruel compassion: Psychiatric control of society's unwanted*. John Wiley & Sons.

Thompson, P. (2000). *The secrets of the great communicators*. ABC Enterprises.

Yamasaki, P. (2022, August 1). The literary definition of euphemisms, with examples. *Grammarly Blog*. Retrieved from www. grammarly.com/blog/euphemism/

Zinsser, W. (2019). *On writing well: The classic guide to writing nonfiction* (30th Anniversary ed.). Harper Perennial.

4 | THE WINNING HABITS OF SUCCESSFUL AUTHORS

INTRODUCTION

Before settling down to the business of producing a written work suitable for publication, there remains here one more task to complete: notably, to examine the winning habits of successful authors. Since habits, by their nature, are hard to break—especially bad habits—it is important that new writers focus on cultivating good writing habits right from the start.

THE WILL TO WRITE

To succeed as a writer, you must not only *want* to write but have *the will to write*—noting here that the will to *write* is much more than the will to *be a writer*. The will to write is taken here to mean 'not just a desire to write, or an impulse to write, but an *overpowering determination* to write' (McAlpine, 2000, p. 9, emphasis added). To put this another way, if you are really serious about writing, you must have a *passion to write*—almost to the point of being fanatical. As Ray Bradbury (1992, p. 4) points out in *Zen in the Art of Writing*:

> if you are writing without zest, without gusto, without love, without fun, you are only half a writer . . . you are not being yourself. You don't even know yourself. For the first thing a writer should be is—excited.

Passion for writing—like any calling—must, however, also be matched by fortitude. Fortitude is necessary because writing involves struggle, and overcoming struggle requires

DOI: 10.4324/9781003413226-4

commitment, since without commitment, it will be difficult to maintain the will to write.

It is difficult to imagine anything more deadly to a person's aspiration to be a writer than a lack of will, a lack of commitment, apathy, a passionate desire to *avoid* the task. If you do not have a passionate desire—the will—to write, and you lack commitment to engaging in the process of writing, then your aspirations should perhaps be focused elsewhere.

WRITE ABOUT WHAT YOU KNOW

It is much easier to write about what you know than what you do not know. Moreover, if you write about that of which you have only cursory knowledge, your audience will soon recognise this and leave your work vulnerable to criticism.

There is a range of benefits of writing about what you know—including not least that in the realm of the known lie many seeds of thought and ideas. If you know a subject area well, you will be in a much better position to generate critical questions, to advance critical discussion on that subject, and to address any substantive intellectual criticisms that may be directed at your work.

WRITE ABOUT WHAT INTERESTS YOU

The importance of writing about what interests you can never be overemphasised. If you do not write about what interests you and what you find deeply significant and meaningful, it will be difficult to progress, to develop as a writer, and to write meaningfully and in a way that will touch your audience. It will also be difficult to find the motivation and fortitude necessary to go the distance, to travel that long and sometimes tortuous path to success. In short, if you do not write about what you are interested in, it will be difficult for you to develop a writing career.

KEEP A NOTEBOOK

It is always important to be open to and keep track of new ideas and thoughts pertinent to your writing. New ideas and thoughts can often come at the most unexpected (and inconvenient) times, such as when you are having a shower, driving a car, reading a book, watching a movie, having a conversation with a friend or colleague, overhearing someone else's conversation, or about to go off to sleep at night. It is important that these ideas and thoughts are noted down as soon as possible; otherwise, you risk forgetting—and hence, losing—them.

It is good practice to have a designated notebook for writing down ideas and thoughts pertinent to your writing. This notebook should be distinctive or of a favourite colour, have a high-quality texture and carry the title 'Writing notebook' or something similar to reflect its special purpose. In addition, it is useful (and also good practice) to have a number of smaller-sized notebooks that can be accessed easily, such as from your pocket, a handbag or briefcase, or the glove box of your car. Keeping 'work in progress' notes is also a good way of keeping a record of the development of your thoughts and will enable you to assess your development as a writer.

PRACTICE WRITING

Like all skills, writing must be practiced if competence (if not excellence) is to be achieved and sustained. Just as professional tennis players and professional musicians must practice for long hours to perfect their skill, so too must writers. On this point, Ray Bradbury (1992, p. xiii) reminds us:

> Remember that pianist who said that if he did not practice every day *he* would know, if he did not practice for two days, the *critics* would know, after three days, his *audiences* would know . . . . A variation of this is true for writers.

There are many opportunities (both formal and informal) for practicing writing during the course of a day. Those working in academic institutions have a particular advantage in this regard since a significant portion of their working day involves writing (emails, memoranda, reports, manuscripts, research proposals, online course materials, lecture notes, subject guides, and so on).

As stated in the Chapter 1, clinicians in the healthcare sector also spend significant periods of time writing as part of their day-to-day professional duties. Whether writing a short email message or case notes on a patient, or writing a larger work such as a report on a quality assurance matter, these are all wonderful opportunities for practicing the art, craft, and science of writing. Furthermore, it is important to remember that 'Any writing helps you with any other writing' (McAlpine 2000, p. 11).

Learning to write takes practice, and practice takes time. The trick is to be realistic about your writing aspirations and goals, and to be patient as you work your way toward achieving them.

MAKE TIME

One of the biggest complaints by aspiring writers (especially those who are also busy professionals) is that they 'do not have time to write' or, if they do have some time, they are simply too exhausted at the end of the day to focus on the job of writing. There is only one solution to this problem: *make time*. If you are serious about writing, you have to find some way of:

- cultivating and preserving your energy for writing
- taking time out of your busy schedule to write.

Making time for writing and taking 'time out' to write requires *discipline*. The amount of time you need and how regularly you need to schedule your writing time will depend on a number of things, including:

- the nature of the work
- the schedule for completion of the work
- the conditions under which you work best; for example, some people work better under pressure and tend to work more efficiently the less time they have—the more time they have, the more time they waste; in contrast, others need more time and less pressure in order to work productively.

Depending on your writing goals, you may only need to set aside a few hours every day (for example, 2–4 hours), or one or two days per week to write. In some instances (for example, when undertaking a major work), you may need to take time off work for several weeks and possibly even months in order to write. While there is no 'one-size-fits-all' programme for time management, one thing is sure: *you need to set up a writing schedule and commit yourself to it*. A writing schedule must include:

- the identification of specific writing projects
- the number of words required per project
- timelines.

Once you have prepared your writing schedule, place it in a prominent place, such as above your writing desk, so that it is kept before you. Once you have done this, highlight the days each week that you plan to work on your projects and the specific tasks that you have chosen.

Facing the task of writing a work of, for example, 4,000 words in length or 40,000 words in length may seem overwhelming in contexts when time is paramount. One way of putting the task into perspective is to remind yourself that there are 365 days in a year. Once you have completed all the preparatory work for your writing (that is, have searched out all your references and other material relevant to the project), if you can manage to write even 400 words a day, you face the very real prospect of being able to complete a draft of a journal article in ten days and a small book in 40 days. Even if you were to write only 200 words a day, it would be possible, by these calculations, to write *several* journal articles each year, not just one. Beware, however, of setting your daily writing schedule too low. Stephen King (2000, p. 121) argues, for example, that beginning professional writers should write *at least* 1,000 words a day, six days per week; anything less than this, he suggests, and 'you'll lose the urgency and immediacy of your story'.

King's prescription is primarily intended for full-time professional writers. Nonetheless, his advice is pertinent even for causal writers: if you do not write a minimum amount of words each day or week, you risk losing the impetus to write. More seriously for part-time writers, if you stop your daily writing when you have reached your set word limit for the day, rather than when you have exhausted your thoughts and writing on the subject matter at hand, the continuity of your thoughts and the entire writing process can be disrupted. Such disruption can be just as frustrating as not writing at all since often when you resume the task of writing, it feels like you are having to start from the beginning all over again.

One way of avoiding having to go back to your original starting point each time you sit down to write is to *compartmentalise* your writing. For instance, when working on a scholarly article, assign yourself the task of writing a specific section on a specified day designated on your scheduled writing. On day 1, for example, focus exclusively on writing the introduction; on day 2, focus on discussing the first point of your article (your first subheading); on day 3, focus on discussing your second point (second subheading); and so on. On scheduled writing days when you do not feel productive, focus on completing mundane tasks such as formulating a table, typing up your reference list, or reading some additional material and making notes.

Eventually, like the pieces of an exquisitely crafted patchwork quilt, all the completed sections of your work can be placed together as a coherent whole, ready for rereading and editing as a completed manuscript.

Serious writing is like a job and should be seen as such. Once you start it, you must be willing to 'shut the door'. As King (2000, p. 121) advises:

> The closed door is your way of telling the world and yourself that you mean business; you have made a serious commitment to write and intend to walk the walk as well as talk the talk.

DEVELOP A 'GOOD' WRITING STYLE

To succeed as a writer, it is imperative that you develop a good writing style. As stated in Chapter 3, style refers to *your* way of writing and the expression of *your* personality and professional voice as an author. Since this topic has already been considered in the previous chapter, I need only say here that it is imperative that authors continually develop and improve their own writing style.

READ PROLIFICALLY AND ATTENTIVELY

Anybody who is serious about writing must READ. Reading is an essential preparatory stage of the writing process. It is critical for the purposes of gaining information, generating ideas, and generally researching the background to your topic. It also serves the critical purpose of helping you develop your own personal writing style.

It is no coincidence that most successful writers are also avid readers who read *with attention*. This is because, as Stephen King (2000, p. 114) explains, 'Reading is the creative center of a writer's life'. It enables writers to get a sense of style and to constantly refine (and redefine) their own work. He also cautions, 'If you don't have time to read, you don't have the time (or the tools) to write. Simple as that'.

When you finish a manuscript, set it aside. There inevitably comes a point when you can do nothing further to a work and it is time to submit it to a journal or a commercial publisher (whichever is relevant) for review. When that point comes, it is also time to move on to the next project. Sit down and start writing the next article or book or whatever else it is that you have scheduled to write. In this way, you will maintain your momentum as a writer.

BE AN EXCELLENT RESEARCHER

To undertake research is to conduct a systematic investigation to establish 'facts' or to collect information on a subject. A professional or an academic article or book will only be as good as the search and research that has been undertaken to inform it. When preparing to write a work, you need to search for, think about, and collate information in a manner that ultimately leaves you and your readers feeling that no rock has been left unturned. Furthermore, always collect more information than you need. There is a common saying in photography circles that a photographer may need to take 100 pictures in order to take the perfect one. Literature searching and researching for an article or a book you are writing involves a similar process: you may need to locate 100 articles in order to find the perfect one—what I call the 'academic gems' for quoting in one's writing. See the subsection 'Preparation' in Chapter 5 for more on this subject.

Have a great filing system

An effective filing system is essential for keeping in order and storing the material you collect to inform and reference your writing. To this end, an eFolder on your computer or a filing cabinet is just as important as a writing desk. How you arrange your filing system is a matter of personal preference and may depend on the nature of the topic or topics you are writing on and the volume of material you have collected. For example, you may wish to organise your material:

- alphabetically according to author surname
- thematically according to subject matter/topics (for example: 'clinical risk management', 'quality assurance', 'research ethics', 'systematic reviews')
- into specific projects (with a separate filing system for each work that is organised in one of the ways previously described).
- using a combination of these methods.

Have a fabulous home library

Every writer needs their own professional library. Writers need to visit bookshops and online resources as frequently as they visit supermarkets to check out what is on the shelves (both material and virtual) and to make purchases as their interests and needs require.

Not all good books and other print resources are available in libraries or online, and sometimes it is only by purchasing books that you maintain ready access to the thoughts and ideas that are contained within them. Further, when writing books, there is something inspiring about being surrounded by them.

The number of books you should have will depend on your interests, finances, home storage capacity, and passion for books. The celebrated Brazilian author Paulo Coelho (author of *The Alchemist* (1988), *Veronika Decides to Die* (1999), and numerous other titles) reveals that he keeps his library to a maximum of 400 books. His decision to keep such a small collection of books is more for practical than ideological reasons: he came home one day and found all the bookshelves that once housed a much larger collection of books had collapsed onto the floor. He worried at the time that had someone been there they might have been killed (Arias, 2001, p. 166).

In your home library, ensure you also have a good reference book section that includes the following range of books:

- at least one good dictionary (preferably more); choices include:
  —*Collins English Dictionary* (which reflects Australian, New Zealand, Scottish, Irish, Canadian, South African, East African, West African, Indian, Caribbean, and British regional English)
  —*Oxford English Dictionary* (which reflects Standard English)
  —*Webster's Dictionary* (which reflects American English)
  —*The Macquarie Dictionary* (which reflects Australian English)
- a good thesaurus
- a good book of quotations—for example, *The Times Book of Quotations* (2000, P. Howard, Intro.); *The Oxford Dictionary of Quotations* (Knowles, 2014)
- the latest edition of <u>*The New Fontana Dictionary of Modern Thought*</u> <u>(2000)</u>
- discipline-specific dictionaries (for example, a dictionary of philosophy, dictionary of sociology, dictionary of psychology, and so forth)
- A good style manual for writers (there are many available).

GET FEEDBACK FROM OTHERS

At some stage during the writing process, writers develop a 'blind spot'. On account of being so close to their own work, writers can lose the discrimination necessary for judging and deciding what is and what is not working in their writing. This can result in writers being either *overly critical* of or *overly satisfied with* their work or, more often, somewhere between the two.

It is at this point that feedback from others (for example: colleagues, prospective readers, students, other writers) can be very useful in terms of either:

- reassuring the writer that their work is interesting, informative, reads well, and is near completion—or *is* complete and ready for submission, or
- advising the writer where improvements could be made, such as by expanding a point, strengthening an argument, better signposting an idea, refining a sentence, filling in a knowledge gap, including a key-reference that appears to have been overlooked, removing redundancies, or picking up typographical errors and other errors that even the most accustomed eye can miss—or *is not* complete and ready for submission.

The key to getting helpful feedback from others is to find a mentor or 'ally reader'. An ally reader is someone who can be trusted:

- *personally*—will have the writer's interests at heart
- *professionally*—has integrity and will not abuse the support relationship to their own professional advantage
- *emotionally*—will not destroy the writer with unconstructive criticism (note, because of the intensely personal

nature of authorship, the craft of writing is an emotionally sensitive process; a writer can thus be made or broken by an insensitive and harsh critic)

- *intellectually*—is competent academically and a 'good thinker'.

In short, and ally reader is someone who is informed, critical, and able to give you sound, reliable, and constructive feedback.

People who will merely tell you how wonderful your writing is or—conversely and discouragingly—how terrible your writing is, should be avoided. It is also important that you have a *trusting relationship* with your mentor or ally reader(s). Trust is important because if you do not trust the people who are giving you feedback it may be difficult to not only accept their advice but to surrender your work to them for feedback at all.

All writers need to get into the habit of utilising ally readers to critique their own work; they can also learn a lot and help other writers by reciprocating the gesture and serving as ally readers themselves.

BE A MENTOR AND COACH TO YOURSELF

Ally readers can provide valuable mentorship to a writer. Ultimately, however, as a writer there is no better mentor than *yourself*. On the issue of self-mentorship, Jack London, author of *The Call of the Wild* (1903) and described as 'an icon of literary success and one of the two or three most popular American writers in the world', wrote: 'in the main I am self-educated; *have had no mentor but myself* [emphasis added] (quoted in Walker & Reesman, 1999, p. ix).

Self-mentorship (or self-coaching) basically involves assisting yourself to achieve your writing goals and develop your writing career. Others can give you support and feedback, and so forth. They cannot, however (and indeed, should not) plan your writing goals, write your work, adopt a lifestyle that enables you to write, submit your work for publication, or accept the rewards and punishments of your work. In several respects, self-mentorship is a necessary precondition to being mentored by others: *a writer must first be willing to help themselves before seeking and accepting the help of others.*

ACCEPT THE REWARDS AND PUNISHMENTS

Like any career, writing has its rewards and punishments. The key to success as a writer is to accept the rewards and punishments *as they come.* In the case of the punishments, it is vital that these are approached with tolerance and patience, and viewed as a valuable opportunity to learn and to develop as a writer and as a person.

Rewards

Undoubtedly among the greatest rewards—if not *the* greatest reward—of writing is seeing the work published and the deep sense of satisfaction you experience when you finally succeed in achieving your writing goal. There is no feeling quite like seeing your work in print. There are, of course, many other rewards:

* receiving positive feedback from reviewers and critics
* learning that your work has 'made a difference' to the lives of others
* having the work nominated for and/or win a literary award
* seeing your work referenced in the work of others and making a significant contribution of knowledge to the field
* receiving a job promotion based on your publication track record

- receiving remuneration (such as royalties)
- being offered other publishing opportunities based on your publication track record
- gaining an international reputation and receiving kudos
- receiving encouragement to keep going.

Punishments

Publishing is a very demanding and competitive activity. And just as its rewards can be rich, its punishment can be painful and demeaning. The punishments of publishing are not insurmountable, however, and in many respects are merely a part of the rites of passage to becoming a successful author. Among the most punishing of experiences for writers are the processes of:

- submission
- rejection
- criticism
- redundancy
- politics of envy.

Submission

When a work is completed, the writer submits the work for publication, or, in other words, *makes a submission* to a chosen publisher. The act of 'submission' can be a very trying and humbling experience for writers. For many, it is tantamount to an act of 'surrender' and literally marks the first step toward 'judgement day' in regard to the merits of the work *and* the credibility of its author. As Gregg Levoy (1997, p. 84) notes, it is perhaps no coincidence that 'the word writers use to describe the act of sending their work out into the world is *submission*. It is indeed a kind of surrender'.

Once a manuscript has been submitted for review, you then have to wait patiently to learn if the work has been accepted for publication or rejected. If there is a delay in the review process, this waiting period can be a challenging time for authors, particularly if they are under pressure to publish a minimum number of articles in any one calendar year, as is the case with academics. A lengthy delay in the review process can also undermine the timely dissemination of the information contained in an article and might even render it obsolete once it goes to press. This, in turn, can impede the capacity of academic authors to disseminate their work in a timely manner and make a significant contribution to the field. It can also undermine an author's ability to achieve their publishing-related performance indicators.

Rejection

The rejection of manuscripts is commonplace and is part of the everyday reality of writing and publishing. If you get a rejection from a publisher, the important thing is *not to take it personally*. Rejections are common even for experienced and successful authors and may not necessarily reflect the quality of the manuscript or the topicality or importance of the work. It may simply be that there is not a profitable market for the work, or it does not 'fit' with a publisher's programme.

Writers have no control over their manuscripts being rejected. They do, however, have control over *how they respond* to the rejections they receive. There is no point getting angry about a rejection notice, since it will not change the outcome. A constructive response is to accept the rejection and 'move on'. Depending on what, if any, feedback has been received, a writer has the options of:

- *accepting* a reviewer's recommendations for amendment, revising the work, and resubmitting it to the same publisher for further review and possible publication
- *rejecting* a reviewer's recommendations for amendment, withdrawing the manuscript from further consideration

and submitting it to a different publisher for review and possible publication

- *partially accepting* a reviewer's recommendations, i.e., making revisions that you accept and providing a rejoinder to the recommendations which you do not agree with or accept.

Either way, it is important to put manuscript rejections into perspective. Although receiving a rejection notification is always disappointing, it does not signal the end of your writing career. If you persevere, develop the habits of other successful writers, remain focused on improving your writing skills and style, and remain determined to achieve your writing goals, chances are you will succeed in getting your work published.

Sometimes, when dealing with a rejection, it can be helpful to talk to or to read about others who have also been through such an experience. The following example of a rejection slip from a Chinese economics journal, quoted in the *Financial Times*, is worth quoting here since it provides a timely reminder to writers to keep the whole process of writing, publishing, and rejection by editors in perspective:

> We have read your manuscript with boundless delight. If we were to publish your paper, it would be impossible for us to publish any work of a lower standard. And it is unthinkable that in the next thousand years we shall see its equal, we are, to our regret, etc.
>
> (cited in Fishman, 2000, p. 129).

Having a manuscript rejected does not mean you have failed in your aspirations to be an author. As Day (1993, p. 8) reminds us,

> Success doesn't happen overnight. A positive attitude, a professional approach and perseverance are usually behind 'sudden' success.

Criticism

Expect that not everyone will agree with or like your work once it is published. Criticism is inevitable. It is important to remember, however, that criticism in the form of *disagreement, disputation,* and *debate* is the *beginning* of our thinking, not its end, and can provide rich fodder for future works. The whole field of philosophy has rested on this premise for centuries and would not have developed to the stage that it has today were it not for a healthy regard for—and acceptance of—the role of disagreement, disputation, and debate in stimulating thought and generating reasoned and defensible arguments for and against certain propositions.

So long as criticism of your work is given within the spirit and legitimate boundaries of academic critique, it can serve the purpose of stimulating further thinking on your subject and of even bringing your work to the attention of a wider audience. What is crucial is *how* the criticism and disagreement is expressed. Obviously, criticism that is personally derogatory or attacks the person rather than the ideas, or which seriously misrepresents a writer's work, is neither appropriate nor acceptable, and may even be libellous (the issue of defamation and libel will be considered further in Chapter 9). It is understandable that a writer would feel hurt and affronted by a personalised attack or a misleading and fraudulent representation of their work. Should this happen to you, always respond with dignity, not in kind. Depending on the seriousness of a criticism (especially if it is defamatory) your options are to either:

- ignore the criticism (thereby denying it the kudos of being worthy of attention)
- publish a patient and considered response to the criticism, pointing out the errors that your critic has made in reading and (mis)representing your work
- place the matter in the hands of your legal representative for mediation and resolution.

Arguably, a more challenging situation for an author is to have his or her work *completely ignored* by critics or other writers in the field. Being ignored, paradoxically, is probably the worst criticism of all since it seems to be saying: *your work is not even worthy of notice, not worthy of attention.*

Redundancy

If you are the author of a book (or books), expect that there will come a time when your work is no longer purchased, photocopied, or cited. Academic books have a relatively short shelf life. The world and contexts in which scientific and practice knowledge is developed is constantly changing, and so it is inevitable that, with time, professional literature once considered to be cutting edge will lose its currency and be regarded as out of date in a relatively short period of time (this is why, with the exception of classical foundational works, some journals require references to be no more than five years old at the time of publication).

Only a very small percentage of academic books stay in print beyond their first print run (that is, are either reprinted as a first edition, or as subsequent revised editions). Once the sales of a book drop below a financially sustainable level, it is no longer a viable business proposition for a commercial publisher. The publisher's options (and contractual rights) are to either let the book go out of print or to decisively withdraw the book from the market and either pulp any remaining copies or remainder what few copies are left at a discount. When this happens, and a publisher notifies you that it has decided not to reprint your book, it is important that you *do not take it personally*. As disappointing as it can be, this is an entirely normal and expected course of events.

Once a book goes out of print, the copyright in the work is normally returned to the author. This means that the author is free to republish the work in whatever form they wish and may approach another company to have the work published as it stands or as a revised edition.

Politics of envy

When you achieve success as an author (and even when you get your first article or book published), understand that not everybody will be as happy and excited as you and your advocates about you having achieved your publishing goals. Unfortunately, people (including those with whom we work closely) do not always respond appropriately or in ways that we might expect in the event of our own or another's scholarly achievements. If your achievements have been the subject of public praise or attention, this can ironically give rise to what Susan Mitchell (2000, p. 98) calls 'the politics of envy'. Reflecting on her own experience as a successful author, newspaper columnist and broadcaster, Mitchell writes:

> When I published my first book, *Tall Poppies*, it became an immediate best-seller. I expected foolishly that my colleagues and, more importantly, my supervisors in the university would be pleased for me and for the reflected success on the institution. Instead, I found not only stony silence on the topic but snide remarks about becoming rich on the book's royalties. And with each successive and successful book, a slow realisation dawned on me that far from being praised for my success in the outside world, I was being punished for it inside the academic world . . . . The unspoken view was that I had received more than my fair share of recognition and praise. My public profile for an academic was already too high.
>
> It took me a long time to come to terms with the fact that my academic colleagues would never give me any recognition for my work.

Mitchell (2000, p. 99) cites the examples of other success-ful authors, including the English writer C.S. Lewis and the Australian playwright David Williamson, who have been the targets of envy on account of their success. Williamson, for example, is reported as admitting that he 'never experienced real vitriol until he became publicly successful in Australia'.

Mitchell (2000, p. 98) contends that 'Public praise, what-ever form it takes, will often bring people in conflict with other people'. Hidden at the base of this conflict, she suggests, is *envy*. On the question of how do deal with the politics of envy, the short answer is simply: *ignore it*. Regain your focus and get on with the business of writing and furthering your career as a successful author.

BE PROFESSIONAL

It is important to treat writing as a profession, and for writ-ers to behave like professionals and to present a professional image in the course of their work.

A professional image is best promoted:

- *In person*—by displaying 'good manners' and observing the rules of common courtesy; being respectful; being reliable, such as by attending appointments on time, responding to phone/email/fax messages promptly, submitting manu-scripts on or before specified timelines; and communicat-ing in an approachable and engaging manner.
- *On paper*—by using business cards; using official statio-nery for correspondence; following the conventions of let-ter writing; using an up-to-date curriculum vitae/résumé that is well set out and portrays you as a credible author and someone who is worth investing in; and presenting manuscripts that comply with author guidelines.

Keeping track of your work and ensuring that you do not 'double up' can also enhance your professional image as an author. To avoid doubling up, keep a record of:

- industry contacts (for example, journal editors, acquisition/managing editors, book representatives)
- phone calls and correspondence to prospective publishers
- material/manuscripts submitted
- who material/manuscripts were submitted to
- when they were submitted
- by what date a reply is expected and the date a reply is received
- why, in the event of rejection, a submission is rejected.

HAVE A PLACE TO WRITE

To write effectively, it is critical that you have a designated space to work. Having a designated writing space (that is, your own writing desk and preferably a study or an office) is just as critical to disciplined writing as is working to a writing schedule. As the English novelist and essayist Virginia Woolf wrote so famously in 1929, 'a woman must have . . . a room of her own if she is to write' (Woolf, 1945, p. 6). This advice applies, of course, to all writers. Having a room of your own means that you can have somewhere to go and that, upon entering that domain, you can 'shut the door'—even if it is only for a few hours—and focus entirely on your writing.

DEVELOP MOMENTUM

Develop momentum as a writer and let the force of this momentum do its work. Describing the nature and importance of momentum, Du Mu counsels in Sun Tzu's *The art of war*, 'Roll rocks down a ten-thousand-foot mountain, and they cannot be stopped—this is because of the mountain, not the rocks' (Tzu, 1988, p. 99).

Success often takes on a life of its own; once achieved, like rocks rolling down a mountainside, it cannot be stopped. As motivational literature is fond of pointing out, 'success breeds success'—that is momentum.

CONCLUSION

Writing needs to be approached in a professional and disciplined manner. In order to develop a successful writing career, writers must first *want* to write and should focus primarily on writing about what they know and what is of interest to them. Writers need also to remember that writing and developing a good writing style takes time, practice, and patience. Reading prolifically and attentively, having a good reference library and other resource materials, getting constructive feedback from others, being a 'self-mentor', being prepared to accept the lows as well as the highs of writing and publishing, and maintaining momentum are all critical to achieving one's writing goals.

EXERCISES
1 Outline what winning habits you have and what habits you need to develop if you are to succeed as an author.
2 Prepare a plan for your writing career.

REFERENCES

Arias, J. (2001). *Paulo coelho: Confessions of a pilgrim*. HarperCollins.

Bradbury, R. (1992). *Zen in the art of writing*. Bantam Books.

Coelho, P. (1988). *The illustrated alchemist: A fable about following your dream*. HarperFlamingo.

Coelho, P. (1999). *Veronika decides to die*. HarperCollins.

Day, M. (1993). *The Art of Self-promotion: Successful promotion by writers*. Allen & Unwin in association with the Australia Council.

Fishman, R. (2000). *Creative wisdom for writers*. Allen & Unwin.

King, S. (2000). *On writing: A memoir*. Hodder & Stoughton.

Knowles, E. (Ed.). (2014). *Oxford dictionary of quotations* (8th ed.). Oxford University Press.

Levoy, G. (1997). *Callings: Findings and following an authentic life*. Thorsons, an imprint of HarperCollins.

London, J. (1903). *Call of the wild*. Macmillan Co.

McAlpine, R. (2000). Develop the will to write. In R. McAlpine (Ed.), *Nine winning habits of successful authors: Tips, tales and inspiration from 44 popular novelists* (pp. 9–11). CC Press.

Mitchell, S. (2000). *Be bold! And discover the power of praise*. Simon & Schuster.

The New Fontana Dictionary of Modern Thought. (2000). *The new fontana dictionary of modern thought*. HarperCollins.

The Times Book of Quotations. (2000). *The times book of quotations* (P. Howard, Intro). HarperCollins.

Tzu, S. (1988). *The art of war* (T. Cleary, trans). Shambhala.

Walker, D., & Campbell Reesman, J. (Eds.). (1999). *No mentor but myself: Jack London on writing and writers* (2nd ed.). Stanford University Press.

Woolf, V. (1945). *A room of one's own*. Penguin Books.

5 | PRODUCING A WORK

INTRODUCTION

Once you have formulated your mission as a writer, prepared your writing schedule, and attended to the 'environmental' issues of writing space, writing tools, and so forth, there comes the task of actually crafting a piece of work—the doing.

Regardless of your field, the topic you are writing on, the level at which you are writing, the proposed length of the work, your intended audience, or your publishing timelines, the act of writing fundamentally involves the following active processes:

1 generating ideas and choosing a topic
2 being clear about what you are setting out to do
3 researching thoroughly and reading widely about the subject
4 examining carefully both your own and others' thinking on the subject
5 allowing your ideas to grow and take shape
6 formulating an outline of what you are going to write
7 engaging in the physical act of writing, structuring the work, and preparing a first draft
8 reviewing and revising the first draft (and where relevant, subsequent drafts) of the work
9 deciding to stop
10 completing the final copy of the work
11 submitting the work for peer review and publication.

THE ACTIVE PROCESS OF WRITING

A good way to make a start and to begin writing productively is to write a brief article such as a case study, a case scenario, a policy brief, or an opinion article on an issue about which you feel strongly and in which you would like others to become interested and potentially take action (for an example of the 'Author Instructions' and editorial requirements pertinent to writing these kinds of articles, visit https://routledgeopenresearch. org/for-authors/article-guidelines/). In pursuing these options, it is important to remember that not all 'good' writing is or has to be the kind of *scholarly* writing that is generally written exclusively for peer-reviewed academic journals. Some very good writing can also be done for and is found in, for example, the correspondence and critical commentary sections of professional journals and other related mass-circulation media (for example, campus and industry magazines, newspapers, and newsletters). Mass-circulation media outlets are always looking for material and are generally receptive to receiving good short articles. The question is: how to start? The short answer is to first, 'Decide what you want to do. Then decide to do it. Then do it' (Zinsser, 2019, p. 285).

WRITING A PERSUASIVE COMMENTARY, EDITORIAL, OR OPINION PIECE

Writing in healthcare domains is not just about communicating ideas; it is also fundamentally about persuading people to accept those ideas and, where applicable, to act on them to achieve some practical purpose. If writing in health professional contexts were not about questioning and challenging the status quo and 'making a difference', there would be little point to it.

Peter Thompson (1998, p. 5) explains that one of the great masters of persuasive communication was the ancient Greek philosopher Aristotle. Indeed, Aristotle's principles of persuasive speech or rhetoric continue to be taught today and 'remain the foundations of modern persuasion'.

According to Aristotle, people can be persuaded by direct evidence or by the use of:

- *ethos* (a speaker's character)
- *logos* (a speaker's reasoned argument)
- *pathos* (the speaker's passion).

(Thompson, 1998, p. 7)

More simply, as Thompson (1998, p. 8) explains, 'being persuasive is really about speaking from your heart, your head and your soul'. Drawing on Aristotle's principles of rhetoric, Thompson (1998, pp. 18–19) believes that the key to persuasive communication is to structure a speech or a presentation according to the following prototype five-point plan:

1 *Bait (exordium)*—A story or statement which arouses audience interest.
2 *Problem or question (narratio)*—You pose a problem or question that has to be solved or answered.
3 *Solution or answer (confirmatio/probatio)*—You resolve the issues which have been raised.
4 *Pay-off or benefit (peroration)*—You state specific advantages to each member of the audience of adopting the course of action recommended in the solution or answer.
5 *Call to action (peroratio)*—You state the concrete actions which should follow your presentation.

An example of how this five-point plan could be used to structure and plan an article on a topic relevant to healthcare is as follows:

Topic—Patients' rights to informed consent and 'do not attempt resuscitation (DNAR)' directives

1 *Bait*—Patients in our public hospitals are being made the subjects of DNAR directives without their knowledge or consent.

2 *Problem*—This situation involves a fundamental violation of patients' rights to be informed and to decide about their care and treatment options.

3 *Solution*—Policies and guidelines on the processes and procedures for prescribing and initiating DNAR directives need to be devised and implemented in the public hospital system.

4 *Pay-off*—Adopting sound DNAR policies and guidelines is good clinical risk management and will help to prevent the withholding or implementation of resuscitation procedures against a patient's will, and spare the hospital and staff from becoming subject to serious complaint and possible litigation.

5 *Call to action*—Develop sound DNAR policies and guidelines for implementation in the public hospital system.

A useful variation of the five-point plan is Thompson's (1998, pp. 26–27) four-point plan, which is structured as follows:

1 *Situation*—The situation is designed to be a brief synopsis or overview of conditions that are already well known to the audience, which sets the focus of the article. Do not create disagreement at this stage.

2 *Complication*—Identify a complication or problem that threatens the viability of the status quo outlined in the situation. The complication may answer one of the following questions:
- what has changed?
- what has happened?
- what is new?
- what is different now?

- what has upset the way things were?
- what has gone wrong?

3 *Question*—The problem identified in the complication leads to the formation of a question. For example:
- what can be done?
- what choices do we have?
- how can we succeed?
- how do we proceed?

4 *Answer*—The answer or hypothesis takes up the bulk of the article and is a detailed response to the issue raised in the question.

An example of how this four-point plan could be used to structure and plan an article on a topic relevant to healthcare is as follows:

1 *Situation*—People suffering from mental illness and other mental health problems are among the most stigmatised, discriminated against, marginalised, disadvantaged, and vulnerable members of society.

2 *Complication*—Although much has been done to improve the status quo, it is evident that a great deal more needs to be done to improve the plight of people with mental illnesses. Unless things are improved, people with mental illnesses will continue to suffer a disproportionate burden of ill health and suffering which, in turn, will have an enormous cost (financial as well as human) for the community and society at large.

3 *Question*—What can be done to improve the status quo? What can be done to improve the plight of people with mental illnesses?

4 *Answer*—We need to overturn the pathology of prejudice and the stigma of difference that is interfering with

processes for achieving social justice for people with mental illnesses. Specifically we need to:

- 'take seriously the perspective of people with mental illnesses' (something that has not been the norm in the past)
- expand the definition of 'who is the same, thus challenging the exclusory uses of differences'; and
- broaden the definition of difference so that more traits (including previously devalued ones) 'become relevant to the distribution of a particular benefit'

(adapted from Minow, 1990, pp. 95–96).

Whether using the five-point or four-point plan, if a work is to achieve its purpose, discussion will need to be informed by reliable references, examples, and quotes, and it will need to exhibit all the principles of style. It is not enough just to write to a plan; as with any other writing, it is also necessary to have a thorough knowledge and understanding of the subject matter in order to be able to put a plan to effective use.

WRITING SCHOLARLY PHILOSOPHIC WORKS AND CRITICAL ESSAYS

Another way of developing your writing career is to write critical or scholarly philosophic essays on a subject. Scholarly philosophic writing has a rich and distinctive history dating back to ancient times and is commonly used in the fields of philosophy, theology, and law. A good example of scholarly work can be found in the influential philosophic works of the ancient Greek philosophers Plato (c. 428—c. 348 BCE) and Aristotle (384–22 BCE); the works of these philosophers have survived to this day and remain in print in different language translations around the world.

Writing a critical essay on a topic of paramount interest can be a good way of starting your writing career, especially if you have not had the opportunity to undertake empirical research on which to publish a report in a peer-reviewed journal. Scholarly inquiry can also serve as a precursor to identifying a subject for investigative research and writing a research application. Thus, it is worthwhile here to explain a little about what philosophic inquiry is and the nature of scholarly philosophic writing.

The tenets of philosophic inquiry and scholarly writing

It is generally recognised within the field of analytical philosophy that a substantial portion of philosophic inquiry is scholarly research. Some knowledge cannot be discovered or developed by empirical research. As the North American philosopher Thomas Nagel (1987, p. 4) explains:

> Philosophy is different from science and from mathematics. Unlike science it doesn't rely on experiments or observations, but only on thought. And unlike mathematics it has no formal methods of proof. It is done just by asking questions, arguing, trying out ideas and thinking of possible arguments against them, and wondering how our concepts really work.

Philosophic inquiry is appropriate for generating new knowledge not obtainable via empirical research. Unlike empirical research, however, philosophic inquiry has no distinctive method (Nielsen, 1987; Emmet, 1968). If there is a method peculiar to philosophy, it is fundamentally that 'of stating one's problem clearly and of examining its various proposed solutions critically' (Emmet, 1968, p. 20). Thus, quoting again from Thomas Nagel (1987, pp. 4–5):

The center of philosophy lies in certain questions which the reflective human mind finds naturally puzzling, and the best way to begin the study of philosophy is to think about them directly. . . . The main concern of philosophy is to question and understand very common ideas that all of us use every day without thinking about them. A historian may ask what happened at some time in the past, but a philosopher will ask, 'What is time?' A mathematician may investigate the relations among numbers, but a philosopher will ask, 'What is a number?' . . . Anyone can ask whether it's wrong to sneak into a movie without paying, but a philosopher will ask, 'What makes an action right or wrong?'

The structure of a scholarly philosophic work

Writing a philosophic work essentially involves writing a defence thesis. The word *thesis* is a Greek word that literally means 'a thing placed'. In the case of a defence thesis, the thing placed is *a proposition*.

Writing a defence thesis provides writers with a wonderful opportunity to take a stand or a position on something, and to develop their ideas in a focused, systematic, thorough, and precise way. Although the ultimate aim is to show there are better reasons for accepting than rejecting the position taken, philosophic writing is generally regarded as being more substantive than mere rhetoric (as discussed earlier), the main difference being that *persuasion* is achieved by carefully considered and reasoned (sound and logical) argument and counterargument, not overblown rhetoric (Seech, 2009).

Scholarly philosophic writing is, by its nature, *argumentative*. It begins with a proposition and then proceeds by expounding 'arguments' in defence of the claim. This process tends to include the articulation not only of arguments *for* the proposition, but the consideration of and response to possible counterarguments to the views expressed. Although it may not be possible to 'prove' a defence thesis, the writer can neverthe-less provide good reasons why a clear-thinking person ought to accept them (Seech, 2009; Watson, 1992).

In scholarly philosophic work, the thesis or proposition is really an 'ultimate conclusion'; and the body of the discussion is really the 'body of evidence' supporting that conclusion (Seech, 2009; Watson, 1992). This body of evidence is comprised primarily of literature sources as well as 'thought experiments' and reasoned arguments.

It should be noted that the term 'argument' as used in philosophic inquiry has a discipline-specific meaning. Specifically, a philosophic argument works by linking a set of statements (called premises) constructed to lead to a conclusion. For a conclusion to be valid, it must follow from its premises. In the following example, for instance, you can see that the conclusion 'Socrates is mortal' is fundamentally linked to and follows directly from the premises that 'All men are mortal' and that 'Socrates is a man':

Premise 1—All men are mortal.
Premise 2—Socrates is a man.
Conclusion—Socrates is mortal.

In order to 'collapse' an argument (by showing it to be false and thereby destroying the case), a critic would need to show (by providing evidence) either that the premises were false and/or that the conclusion does not follow from the premises. For example, in order to collapse the preceding argument, a critic would need to show that either:

1 not all men are mortal (present the example of even one man who is living forever)
2 Socrates is not a man (Socrates could, for example, be a fish)

3   Socrates is immortal (the conclusion does not follow from the premise, for example, where it has been shown that Socrates is not a man but a rare immortal fish).

Now to use a more realistic example, consider the following argument:

Premise 1—People should always have high-fibre cereals for breakfast
Premise 2—X is a high-fibre cereal
Conclusion—All people (including myself) should eat X for breakfast.

In order to collapse this argument, or to show that it is not 'true', a critic would need only to show (with scientific evidence) that:

Against premise 1—Not all people should, in fact, have high-fibre cereals for breakfast (for example, those who are fasting and those who, for reasons of illness, cannot tolerate high-fibre foods)
Against premise 2—X is not, in fact, a high-fibre cereal (it may have been mistakenly thought to be a high-fibre cereal)
Against the conclusion—It is not the case that all people (including myself) should eat X for breakfast.

Unfortunately, it is not possible within the scope of this present work to provide an in-depth discussion on the elements, form, content, and general nature of philosophic reasoning and argument, and its application in healthcare scholarship. These issues are discussed comprehensively in *Writing Philosophy Papers* by Zachary Seech (2009) and in *Writing Philosophy: A Guide to Professional Writing and Publishing* by Richard A

Watson (1992), both of which are still in print, with the latter also available in some university library eBook collections (via EBSCOhost). In the space remaining, however, it is appropriate to outline the general structure of a philosophic work and dispel some of the popular misconceptions and misunderstandings that still surround scholarly philosophic writing in healthcare domains.

Like all writing, scholarly writing has a beginning, a middle, and an end. The opening paragraph to a scholarly work should precisely state the claim or 'point of contention' to be defended in the body of the work and include an outline of how it will be defended. The body of the work (the main discussion) should present the 'evidence' (arguments and counter-arguments) supporting the point of contention. Finally, the conclusion should summarise what has been achieved. In essence, the conclusion should do little more than 'mirror' the opening paragraph: it should briefly restate the claim (point of contention), review the main arguments advanced in support of it, and generally confirm delivery of what was promised in the opening paragraph (Seech, 2009). As a general rule, no *new* material should be introduced in the conclusion. If the ideas in a conclusion have not been defended in the body of the work, *they should not be included.*

Before commencing a scholarly work, it is advisable to plan or outline the basic structure of your paper. Devising such a plan will help you to:

- focus, organise, and order your thinking
- check and track the logic and coherency of the arguments you are planning to advance in support of your proposition
- help you to 'keep on track' and not get distracted by issues that are tangential to your topic (Seech, 2009; Watson, 1992).

Prototype plan for structuring a scholarly philosophic paper

The following is a prototype plan for structuring a scholarly philosophic paper.

1 *Opening paragraph*
   a Statement of the 'point of contention' or claim to be defended
   b Outline of the main points or arguments to be advanced in support of the claim made:
      i point 1 (also serving as a 'signpost' to the first subheading)
      ii point 2 (also serving as a 'signpost' to the second subheading)
      iii point 3 (also serving as a 'signpost' to the third subheading).
2 *Body of the discussion*
   a point 1 (subheading)
   b point 2 (subheading)
   c point 3 (subheading).

(*Note*: Discussion under the respective subheadings may be broken up under further sub-subheadings. Counter-arguments can be presented as sub-subheadings under these points or under a separate subheading, whichever is appropriate).

3 *Conclusion*
   a Restatement of the point of contention
   b Restatement of the mains points advanced in support of the point of contention:
      i point 1
      ii point 2
      iii point 3.

An example of how this prototype plan might be used to outline the content and approach of an article on a specific healthcare topic is as follows:

Topic—Health professionals reported for the misconduct of child maltreatment: ethical issues for disciplinary panels

1 *Opening paragraph*
    a Point of contention—Regulating authorities should adopt a formal policy position of 'zero tolerance' towards health professionals found to have abused children and should impose the maximum penalty of deregistration in cases when allegations have been sustained.
    b Outline of the main points to be advanced in support of the claim made:
        i child maltreatment is professional misconduct of a *serious nature at the upper end of seriousness*
        ii child maltreatment by health professionals constitutes a violation of conduct standards otherwise expected by the public
        iii regulating authorities have a primary obligation to protect the public interest, not the professionals who have offended against children
        iv misconduct of a serious nature at the upper end of seriousness warrants the severest of sanctions: *deregistration*.
2 *Body of the discussion*
    a First subheading—'Child maltreatment as professional misconduct of a serious nature'
    Sub-subheadings:
        i 'The nature of child maltreatment'
        ii 'The nature of professional misconduct'
        iii 'The constituents of misconduct of a 'serious nature' at the 'upper end of seriousness'.

b Second subheading—'Professional conduct standards'
Sub-subheadings:
  i 'Nature and purpose of professional conduct standards'
  ii 'Standards of professional conduct expected by the public'.
c Third subheading—'Health professional regulating authorities and protection of the public interest'
Sub-subheadings:
  i 'Protecting the public interest'
  ii 'Public trust and protecting the good reputation and standing of the profession'
  iii 'Professional misconduct of a serious nature and forfeiting the right to practice as a professional'
  iv 'Nature and purpose of a "zero tolerance" position'
  v 'Moral and professional imperatives of adopting a "zero tolerance" position and de-registering health professionals who have maltreated children'.

3 *Conclusion*—Regulating authorities have a responsibility to adopt a formal policy position of 'zero tolerance' towards health professionals found to have abused children and impose the maximum penalty of deregistration in cases were allegations have been sustained. This is because:

a Child maltreatment is professional misconduct of a *serious nature.*
b Child maltreatment by health professionals constitutes a violation of conduct standards otherwise expected by the public.
c Regulating authorities have a primary obligation to protect the public interest, not the professionals who have offended against children.
d By deregistering health professionals who have maltreated children, regulating authorities will send a message to the public and to the profession that the

abuse of children is not acceptable and that health professionals have a special obligation to protect children and to take appropriate action when the interests of children are violated by people in a professional and trusted position.

WRITING EMPIRICAL RESEARCH ARTICLES

Writing an investigative empirical research article—that is, an article in which the findings of either a quantitative or qualitative research study are presented—is arguably more straightforward than writing scholarly philosophic works. Depending on the journal in which the work is published, empirical research articles are generally structured in keeping with the following main sections (identified under 'Author Instructions' in https://routledgeopenresearch.org/for-authors/article-guidelines/), noting there may be some variations, depending on the journal):

1 Author
2 Title
3 Abstract
4 Key words
5 Main body
   • Introduction
   • Methods
   • Results
   • Discussion/conclusion
6 Data availability
7 Limitations of the study
8 Author contribution
9 Competing interests
10 Grant information
11 Ethics approval

12 Acknowledgements (where due)
13 Supplementary material
14 References and footnotes
15 Figures and tables (if used)
16 Images (if used)

Whether reporting the findings of a quantitative or qualitative study, the opening paragraph in the Introduction section should contain a poignant opening sentence to 'hook' the reader. Unless there is a separate subheading signalling a discussion on the background to the study, the opening paragraph usually provides an overview of the research study including:

- information on the background to and rationale for the study
- the research question(s)
- the aims of the study.

Under the 'Methods' subheading, attention is given to discussing:

- the theoretical underpinnings of the study
- the description of the sample
- the means of accessing the sample
- data collection and analysis
- limits of the study
- a statement confirming ethics approval and compliance with prescribed research ethics standards.

The presentation of results/findings and their discussion will depend on the nature of the study and, crucially, the word limit set by a receiving journal. Findings are usually presented and discussed in the form of a succinct synopsis rather than as an elaborate exhaustive narrative. The discussion section provides a discussion of the answers to the research questions; if there is no sub-headed conclusion to the article, the discussion in this section generally concludes with a recommendation for further research and, where appropriate, a call for the practical application of the findings such as in the form of a practice or policy change. Statements in a conclusion are typically crafted along the lines of possible areas or issues warranting further investigation.

Although the structure of empirical research articles is less complicated than philosophic papers, writers still need to take care in crafting their work. As with any scholarship, the background to an empirical study, the processes used for undertaking the study, and the study's findings all need to be presented and discussed in a logical, salient, coherent, and defensible manner. The strategies of philosophic writing can be particularly helpful in this regard, particularly when providing a critical discussion of the findings. Even though the techniques of philosophic writing and reasoning are not the primary 'methods' used in empirical research articles, they nonetheless have an important adjunct role to play.

When relevant, the use of tables and figures need to be pertinent and presented clearly in the article.

WRITING FOR NEWSLETTERS

Writing for a profession's or an organisation's newsletters can provide another valuable opportunity to develop your skills as a writer. Although newsletters tend to be informal in style, writing articles for inclusion in them should still be approached with diligence, discipline, and care. A newsletter that is badly produced and contains 'bad' writing could prove a disaster for the organisation or group sponsoring it and the writers contributing to it.

The primary purpose of a newsletter is to promote communication between an organisation or a special interest group and its constituents (Baverstock, 2002). For example, university newsletters are produced to foster communication between the organisation's:

- industry partners
- staff
- current students
- alumni
- other academic colleagues, both within and outside of the university.

Other key purposes served by the production of a newsletter are to:

- *connect* with constituents and to foster in them a sense of community and belonging
- *inform* and keep constituents up to date with the latest happenings and issues of mutual interest
- *involve* constituents by giving them an opportunity to respond to and to participate in certain events and activities promoted in the newsletter (including contributing articles)
- *activate* constituents by putting out a 'call to action'.

Writing in newsletters tends to be *conversational* in style. In using a conversational style of writing, however, just as much attention needs to be paid to the elements and principles of style (see Chapter 3 of this book) as with scholarly and other creative non-fiction writing.

Successful newsletter writing and production have a number of features in common. In summary, 'good' newsletter writing is:

- *current*—and preferably a 'step ahead' of other outlets
- *concise*—most contributions should normally be no longer than 350–400 words in length

- *accurate*—information contained in an article should be accurate, valid, and reliable; if fraudulent or inappropriate claims are made in the material published, this can be very damaging not only to the writer but also to the newsletter and to the organisation or group producing it
- *informative*—shares information that is of interest, is pertinent, and meets readers 'need to know'.

GENERAL ADVICE ON PRODUCING A WORK

Whether writing for publication in a professional journal, a book, a blog, a newspaper or a newsletter, careful attention should always be paid to the following processes.

Choosing a title

Choosing a title for a work can be an exasperating experience for a writer. One day you might think you have the perfect title only to change your mind the next and deem it trivial and boring. Regardless, it is important that when you start writing an article or book, you at least have a *working title* for the work. Once you have a working title, then you can start looking for the 'perfect title'—which can take some time. Susan Page (1998, p. 24) argues, controversially, that in your quest for the 'fabulous title', you should sit down and write no less than 30 titles in one sitting! Once you have a title and have a sense that it is right, ask others for their opinion and gauge their reactions.

The title of a work should:

- convey to the reader what the work is about
- provide this information at a glance (bearing in mind that readers often scan bookshelves looking for titles relevant to their interests and will pick up only those that catch their eye)
- convince the reader the work is 'for them'.

According to Page (1998, p. 18) a good title should accomplish most if not all of the following tasks:

- instantly say what the work is about
- pique our curiosity
- be distinctive
- be memorable
- be positive
- feel on target, exciting, and compelling *to the author.*

A title should also be descriptive, not metaphorical, and contain key words that will ensure it is noticed and located in the appropriate citation indexes. For example, a paper entitled 'The tea-bag phenomenon' (which is about 'infusing' the findings of healthcare research into practice) will probably not be noticed as readily as it might otherwise be if it contained keys words more appropriate to its subject matter and content such as 'translating research into practice'.

Other helpful tips in crafting a title are:

- avoid words that can be spelled in different ways
- make the title easy to remember
- avoid titles that begin with *How to* . . . (books in print contain over 6,000 titles that begin with these words)
- include subtitles (these give you the chance to add more information to a title and to hook a potential reader.

(adapted from Page, 1998, pp. 21–22)

Preparation

Critical to any writing process is the level of preparation that is undertaken before embarking on the work. Preparation includes not just undertaking a pertinent or exhaustive literature search and review, but also thinking deeply about the topic, being open to and exploring new ideas (from all manner of sources, including informal and incidental sources), and generally ordering your thoughts on the topic. It also involves deciding 'what single point you want to leave in the reader's mind' (Zinsser, 2019, p. 43) and working diligently to uphold all the principles of style to enable you to make that point powerfully, impressively, and persuasively.

The quality of a work will always depend on the quality of the information contained within it—whether it is accurate, pertinent, salient, and complete—not merely on the manner of its presentation. A work could, for example, be technically perfect yet utterly lifeless and unimpressive. When preparing to write a work, you should search for, think about, and collate information in a manner that ultimately leaves you feeling that 'no rock has been left unturned' and ensures that the completed work leaves the reader with that feeling, too.

Literature reviews

Sometimes writers preparing literature reviews for a research thesis or report write to show *what they have read*, rather than to provide an auditable trail of the intellectual path they have followed. When writing a literature review, it is important that you consider whether the literature you have reviewed provides evidence for the points you are advancing. If not, do not include it in your final report/manuscript.

Writing an abstract

An abstract is a short summary or a condensed version of a piece of writing such as a journal article, research proposal, or report (the journal abstract equivalent for a book is normally its Preface). An abstract may range in length from 50–300 words, depending on the publication or research application document in which it will appear.

Abstracts are commonly used in electronic abstract databases such as EBSCOhost, PROQUEST CENTRAL, WEB

OF SCIENCE, SCOPUS, MEDLINE CENTRAL, and CINAHL, and hence are widely disseminated. When writing an abstract, it is therefore important to keep in mind its fundamental purpose—namely, to allow other researchers to scan quickly through the latest professional publications to source information that is relevant to their work. For example, it is possible to scan up to 600 abstracts in a few hours when undertaking a literature search for a journal article or other publication. Being able to scan the abstracts over such a relatively short period of time (much shorter than it would take to read 600 articles) can speed up the research process and enable the writer to establish very quickly whether their thoughts, ideas, and work are up to date, relevant, original, and critical.

When crafting an abstract, the principles of Aristotle's rhetoric (see the section 'Writing a persuasive commentary, editorial, or opinion piece' earlier in this chapter) apply since, in essence, you are trying to *sell* your article or report to prospective readers. The abstract should have a beginning, middle, and an end; include key words; and provide a poignant snapshot of what the broader work is about. It may contain similar or even the same words used in an opening paragraph.

What you write will ultimately depend on the economy of words available to you. Whether writing 50 words or 300 words, however, extreme discipline—and style—is required.

In addition to abstracts, journals require a list of key words. The purpose of listing key words is to enable indexers and search engines to locate relevant papers that have been published on a given topic. Key words can be generated from a 'good' abstract by using the PubMed search tool 'MeSH on demand' (https://meshb.nlm.nih.gov/MeSHonDemand). To use this tool, simply cut and paste the abstract into the search box and click 'search', and key words will be generated.

Crafting the introduction

In several respects, the most important sentence and the most important paragraph of a work is the *first one*. This is because the first sentence and the paragraph that it leads into serves fundamentally as the 'hook' to prospective readers. If readers are not engaged immediately and if there is no incentive to read on, they will simply not continue.

When crafting your opening paragraph to a work, and the paragraphs following it, keep in mind the following principles:

- the lead sentence must capture the reader immediately
- the lead 'must provide hard details that tell the reader why the piece was written and why they ought to read it' (what is in it for them?)
- coax the reader along the way
- tell a story
- add an element of surprise (for example, use something unexpected; the contrapuntal device can achieve this)
- when you are ready to stop, just stop.

(adapted from Zinsser, 2019, pp. 45–52)

The use of headings and subheadings

Headings and subheadings are titles that serve to delineate subsections of a work. The main purpose of headings and subheadings is to provide 'signposts' to the reader so they know in which direction the information is heading.

In books, headings become the *table of contents* which can also serve as an 'easy find' index to the work (see, for example, the table of contents to this work). Writing out the headings and subheadings of a work (whether as a table of contents for a book, or as an outline for a journal article or book chapter) can give the writer an overall sense of the coherency of the work and where certain sections may need to be relocated to ensure a better progression of the ideas being advanced. To be effective signposts, titles and subtitles need to be:

- clear about what is contained in the section or subsection
- short
- distinctive
- relevant (deliver what it says it will)
- eye-catching
- enticing to the reader.

The 'Matrioshka principle'

All works should have a clearly distinguishable beginning, middle, and end. In addition, each subsection and sub-subsection of a work should likewise have a distinguishable beginning, middle, and end. It should be possible with a well-written piece of work to pick up any section of the work and, upon reading it, get a sense of and feel informed about both its parts as well as its whole. Like the classical Russian nesting doll (the *Matryoshka*, or the anglicised variant *Matrioshka*) which is characteristically comprised of *a doll nestling within a doll nestling within a doll*, and where each of the smaller dolls is a perfect or near-perfect replica of the immediate larger doll in which it is found, each subsection of a discussion should stand as a complete 'mini-discussion' in a larger work—that is, as *a discussion within a discussion within a discussion*. For teaching and writing purposes, I have called this the 'Matrioshka principle of writing'.

Unfettered writing

When embarking on your writing, do not unduly limit or constrain yourself. Nothing can be more constraining to your creative thinking and writing than feeling fettered by a word limit or even by a writing plan. It is more productive to write freely and then radically edit a work to comply with a word limit than it is to write tightly to a word limit from the beginning. Similarly, when writing to a plan, it is better to exhaust your thoughts—even those that might be tangential to your work—than it is to constrain your thinking. Ideas and commentary that are tangential to your work can always be edited out later. In the interests of writing an innovative and benchmark work, 'Think broadly about your assignment . . . . Push the boundaries of your subject and see where it takes you' (Zinsser, 2019, p. 174). If experiencing writer's block, then first engage in 'free writing' (discussed in Chapter 6), then—once you have organised your ideas and thoughts—engage with the writing process and write freely.

Staying on track

When writing, it is always tempting to include and discuss issues that, while interesting, are not strictly relevant to the key point or points you are trying to make and emphasise. An important and general rule for writers is: *keep on track*. To assist you in deciding what is and what is not strictly relevant, apply the following rule: *if the information and/or references you are considering provide necessary support or background to a point you are trying to make, then include the material; if not, exclude it.*

Crafting the conclusion

Crucial to any writing is deciding where, when, and how to conclude it. Often a work will tell you where it wants to stop, in that the ending just 'feels right' (Zinsser, 2019, pp. 43–51). When the ending comes, it is always important that readers have something to 'go away with'.

Pay careful attention to crafting the conclusions of your work. Just as the first sentence should function as a hook to *read on*, the last sentence should also function as a hook to *read further* on the subject, to take action, or to recommend the work to others. Finish on an inspiring note. At the very least, leave the reader with a sense that the work and its conclusion were worth reading. Better still leave the reader with a powerful idea, an image, a taste, or a desire to question and to act.

Bibliographies and reference lists

Novice writers are sometimes confused about the nature, purpose, and the differences between a bibliography and a reference list, and which they should use. Your decision to use a reference list or a bibliography will have as much to do with the conventions and editorial requirements of a journal or publisher as it will with your own personal preference. Most journals require reference lists; some journals also prescribe an upper limit on the number of references that can be used. In the case of book publishing, depending on word-limit requirements, some may advocate the use of either a reference list or a bibliography, or a combination of both.

The essential difference between a reference list and a bibliography is as follows:

- a *reference list* includes only those works that have been cited or *quoted directly* in the text of a work
- a *bibliography* includes all works that have been *consulted* or *read* during the course of writing the text, including those that have *not* been cited or quoted from directly.

When deciding whether to include a reference list or a bibliography in your publications, consider the following:

- the purpose of either a reference list or a bibliography is to leave an 'audit trail' so that readers can locate and gain access to the original works to which you have referred in the body of your work

- *always* include a full list of the works you have quoted from or used in preparing your publication
- including an accurate list of all the works you have read—and which have influenced and/or informed your writing—assures readers of the integrity of your work and protects you against committing plagiarism
- editorial requirements and prescribed word limits may limit your options: you may have to include *either* a bibliography *or* a reference list depending on what has been prescribed by the publisher.

CONCLUSION

Producing a work for publication (whether a journal article, a book, a blog, a newspaper commentary, or an item for a newsletter) requires careful planning and thought. It also requires disciplined attention to drafting, redrafting, and conducting a final edit of the work before submitting it for publication. Deciding when to stop can sometimes be as difficult as getting started. Often, however, the work draws to a 'natural' conclusion leaving the writer with a feeling of 'Ah, ha—that's it! It's finished!'.

EXERCISES

1 With reference to Thompson's five-point or four-point plan (see pages 83–86 of this chapter), write a persuasive commentary on a professional issue that is presently of concern to you and your colleagues.
2 Submit your commentary for publication in an appropriate professional journal or other publication.
3 Based on your commentary, prepare a plan for writing a scholarly article on the issue.

4 Share your commentary and writing plan with your mentor for feedback.
5 Commence researching and reviewing the literature in preparation for writing your scholarly article.
6 Set a writing schedule and commence writing the article.
7 Upon completion, submit the manuscript to an appropriate journal for review and publication.

REFERENCES

Baverstock, A. (2002). *One step ahead: Publicity, newsletters and press releases*. Oxford University Press.

Emmet, L. (1968). *Learning to philosophize*. Penguin Books, Harmondsworth, Middlesex.

Minow, M. (1990). *Making all the difference: Inclusion, exclusion, and American law*. Cornell University Press.

Nagel, T. (1987). *What does it all mean? A very short introduction to philosophy*. Oxford University Press.

Nielsen, K. (1987). Can there be progress in philosophy?. *Metaphilosophy*, *18*(1), 1–30.

Page, S. (1998). *How to get published and make a lot of money!*. Piatkus.

Seech, Z. (2009). *Writing philosophy papers* (5th ed.). Wadsworth/ Cengage-Learning.

Thompson, P. (1998). *Persuading Aristotle: The timeless art of persuasion in business, negotiation and the media*. Allen & Unwin.

Watson, R. A. (1992). *Writing philosophy: A guide to professional writing and publishing*. Southern Illinois University Press.

Zinsser, W. (2019). *On writing well: The classic guide to writing nonfiction* (30th Anniversary ed.). HarperPerennial.

6 | TROUBLESHOOTING

INTRODUCTION

During the writing process, all writers—both novice and experienced—will encounter difficulties that they have not encountered before. Whether writing a journal article, a case study, a policy brief, a critical commentary, or a report, questions will arise and challenges will be encountered that need to be addressed. Whether the difficulties encountered are to be regarded as 'serious' will depend largely on the extent to which they:

- interfere with, impede, or obstruct the writing process
- delay unacceptably or even prevent a work from being completed and published, not only on time but at all.

How well writers deal with the challenges they encounter will often depend on their character, how creative they are, how disciplined their thinking is, and how willing and able they are to engage constructively with others who share their interests and perspectives.

While there is no magic recipe for dealing with the various difficulties that writers will inevitably encounter during the course of their writing careers, there are nevertheless some strategies that can be utilised to help prevent some of the more common types of difficulties from occurring—or at least minimise their negative impact should they occur. One strategy is to know about the kinds of problems that can occur, anticipate them at the outset, and have strategies in place to deal with them if and when they are encountered. Following are some examples.

DOI: 10.4324/9781003413226-6

GENERATING IDEAS

For some writers, particularly novice writers, the most difficult task is deciding what to write about and how to generate ideas. Difficulties can be encountered not just in finding topics to write on, but also in generating enough ideas to sustain the writing itself. In contrast, experienced writers may never be short of ideas and are instead faced with the challenge of how to recognise and choose the most salient ideas for their work.

There are a number of strategies that can be used for generating ideas, such as the following:

1   Be curious and learn to *recognise ideas*. Ideas are scattered everywhere, not just in conventional sources (such as libraries, academic books, and journal articles); look for ideas/material everywhere, for example, in:
    - your surveillance of the world/workplace
    - newspapers, magazines, and mass-circulation media
    - visual arts—e.g., film, documentaries
    - conversations (both formal and informal)
    - your social network (family/friends)
    - yourself (for example, personal experiences, responses to the human condition, political outrage)
    - your own publications—'In the body of every article you write lurk the seeds of several more' (Holmes, 1969, p. 20)
    - the publications of others.
      (adapted from Holmes, 1969, pp. 11–21; Zinsser, 2019; Ruggiero, 2015)
2   Always collect more material than you will use. If something attracts your attention, collect it even if you are not sure how or if you will use it. There is nothing quite so frustrating as writing a work and suddenly remembering an anecdote or a quote or a reference, but not remembering its source or how to locate it.

3 Write down your ideas immediately: *keep a notebook and use it*. Then, using the ideas you have noted down, just sit down and *write*.

OVERCOMING WRITER'S BLOCK

'Writer's block' is a colloquial term that is used to describe a situation in which a writer cannot think, cannot write, and as a result cannot move forward in the writing process. It is, quite simply, a dreadful situation in which a writer finds themselves 'stuck' and which, paradoxically, sees the writer spending a large amount of writing time and energy '*not* writing' (Elbow, 1998, p. 14) (Emphasis Original).

Writer's block can occur at any time during the writing process: in the beginning, the middle, and/or at the end of a work. Both inexperienced and experienced writers can experience it.

The causes of writer's block are many, and include:

- *lack of confidence*—in one's own ability to produce the work
- *fear*—of producing a substandard work and what others might think about it (the fear of producing 'nothing but rubbish')
- *panic*—about a looming deadline and whether the work will be completed on time
- *perfectionism*—the desire to produce a word-perfect draft/copy on the first attempt
- *exhaustion*—from working too hard at your usual job and literally being depleted of the energy to think and write.

The best way to overcome writer's block is to:

- avoid being judgemental about the situation and about yourself (accept that it 'just is', and that it will pass)

- avoid censuring or trivialising your work (this is being judgemental and will serve only to further cement your sense of being stuck and your procrastination)
- engage in 'free writing'[1] (no matter how 'blocked' you are feeling, sit down and write without stopping for 10–15 minutes; it does not matter if the writing is good or bad since the whole point of this exercise is *to get writing* and to overcome the block in the process)
- resume the writing project: *get on with it.*

If you are exhausted, all that you may need is some 'space'— that is, a short rest and a temporary break away from the writing process. Sometimes just going for a 20-minute walk can refresh and reinvigorate you. Whatever you decide to do, ensure that you resume writing as soon as possible so that you can get back on track.

DEALING WITH PROCRASTINATION

Procrastination is a form of writer's block and, unresolved, can be just as disruptive to the writing process as writer's block. The causes of procrastination are similar to those that cause writer's block: lack of confidence, fear, perfectionism, exhaustion, and overwork.

The best way to deal with procrastination is to:

- avoid being judgemental about the situation and about yourself (accept that every writer experiences procrastination at some stage during the writing process and that it will pass; say to yourself in a matter of fact way, 'That's me—procrastinating', and let go)
- write a list of the things that you are putting off
- examine the list and assign a priority value to each task, putting the most important first and the least important

last (sometimes, however, starting on and completing a small though unimportant task, like adding a couple of references to your bibliography, can help to break the mood of procrastination since it is one less thing on the list that needs to be done and may be just enough to lessen the 'pressure cooker effect' that is stalling you in your work)

- focus on undertaking the most important and most urgent task first
- take one step at a time; as Maskell and Perry (1999, p. 165) advise:

> Don't allow yourself to feel overwhelmed by the extent of the task—break it down into a series of small steps. Keep each step simple and achievable. Take one step at a time and reward yourself as you complete each step.

- seek assistance (if the task is too difficult, or you have other tasks pressing that others could do, negotiate for some help)
- start writing (putting off the task does not get it done; furthermore, the longer you put it off, the bigger the task seems and the more overwhelming it becomes).

BENEFITS AND CHALLENGES OF CO-AUTHORSHIP

In many academic and professional circles, collaborative writing and co-authorship is the norm and not the exception. Collaborating with other authors both within and outside of your field or discipline can have many benefits, and when one is invited to collaborate on a work, it can feel like a great honour—especially if the invitation has been extended to you in recognition of your standing in the field. Collaborative writing can also pose many challenges, and when one is faced with some of those challenges, it can feel like a great burden.

One of the key benefits of author-collaboration is the sharing of discipline-specific knowledge and experience in a manner that enables:

- the development of new ideas and alternative perspectives on a subject
- improved and deeper understanding of a subject
- the creation of 'new knowledge'
- the development of innovative and productive connections between different and related subject matter
- finding new solutions to old problems and new solutions to new problems
- bridging the gap between theory and practice (particularly in the case of academic–clinician collaborations)
- mentorship of inexperienced writers by experienced authors
- personal development (including the development of interpersonal skills and learning to work productively with others)
- professional development (not least developing multi-disciplinary skills outside of the knowledge and experience of your own discipline).

Another benefit of collaborative writing is that it shares the burden of writing and producing publications to meet academic performance indicators. For instance, collaborating with a team of three or four authors and rotating the primary and associate author responsibilities to reflect the degree of each author's contribution to a work could result in an author participating in three or four peer-reviewed articles per year, instead of just one. Likewise with publishing larger works such as books. A book of 12 chapters written respectively by 12 authors or cooperatively with three collaborating authors is less onerous and arguably more manageable in a busy academic year than publishing a book of 12 chapters written by just one author.

Writing collaboratively also brings with it certain challenges. Collaborative writing can become particularly demanding when disagreement and conflict arises between participating authors. Disagreements and conflicts can occur about such things as the specific sections of a manuscript a contributing author is responsible for, what content should be included and excluded, the order in which contributing authors should be listed on the final manuscript, who should be cited as the lead author, and the like. These issues can arise even when a writing plan has been devised collaboratively and agreed upon (including who should be the lead author) before the project has begun. One reason for these conflicts is that most writers do their thinking and writing simultaneously, and it is not until they actually sit down and write that it becomes clear what it is they are thinking and where their ideas are leading to. Thus, it is not until collaborating writers start their work and share their writing with each other that differences become evident in their:

- intellectual standpoints
- writing skills (in some instances, it may even become evident that a collaborating writer cannot write well)
- writing styles
- work habits
- attitudes toward the work
- priorities assigned to the work
- personalities.

In extreme cases, these differences can result in the authors moving in different directions, to the detriment of the work. Sometimes this can happen even when the collaborating authors have agreed to work with each other on the basis of 'knowing each other' and 'knowing each other's work' prior to the commencement of the collaborative project.

Dealing with disagreement and conflict between collaborating authors can be both difficult and stressful, particularly if it is impeding the progress of the work and the team's ability to meet the contractual timeline for the delivery of the completed manuscript. Professional relationships and reputations are also at stake. For these reasons, it is imperative that conflicts between collaborating authors are resolved quickly and professionally. Strategies for preventing and dealing with a possible breakdown in author-collaborations include:

1 *Choose your co-authorship team carefully in the first place*—remember, we often do not know the people we work with as well as we think, and it is not until we work *closely* with them that we discover their true character and capabilities; remember also that the nature of a person's published work may not necessarily reflect how difficult or easy they are to work with as a collaborating author (this applies whether you are the author inviting collaboration or you have been invited to collaborate with another author).

2 *Complete a detailed plan of the project before commencement of the work*—ensure that all co-participating authors are informed about, are clear about, understand, and agree on the subject of the work, the rationale for writing it, the aims and objectives, the intended audience, the special features and characteristics that would distinguish the work from other similar works, and the word limits, timelines, and each author's specific rights, duties, and responsibilities in regard to the work (*note*: it is wise and in some institutions a mandatory requirement to sign an 'authors agreement' form before commencing a work; this agreement should clarify issues such as intellectual property rights, author responsibilities, the order in which the authors should be

listed on the manuscript, and so forth—much like a book contract). (The issue of author rights and responsibilities will be considered further in Chapter 8 of this book).

3 *Act quickly and decisively to resolve conflict*—if and when there is so much as a *hint* of divisive differences emerging between the authors, work collectively, collaboratively, and professionally to resolve these differences *as soon as possible*; differences that are allowed to fester can become irreconcilable and can place both the team and the work in jeopardy. In cases involving disputes about the order in which co-authors should be cited, it may be necessary to involve a third party (such as a head of department) to mediate the dispute.

4 *Have a back-up plan*—sometimes the differences between one or more authors can become irreconcilable and it might be better, on the basis of a 'cost–benefit' analysis, for the disgruntled author/authors to withdraw from the project; in the event of this happening, make provisions for the writing responsibilities to be shared, where able, among the remaining authors or engage a replacement author to carry out the work.

5 *Learn from the experience*—in the event of an author-collaboration breaking down, conduct a 'root cause' analysis of what went wrong and use the learning gained from conducting this analysis to inform the development and conduct of future collaborative projects.

PROMISES AND PERILS OF COMMISSIONED WRITING

On occasion, a healthcare professional or academic might be commissioned by a professional organisation, a government department, an independent publisher, or some other entity to produce a 'special work' such as a book, a manual, or a report on a designated topic for a clearly specified purpose and for a specific audience. Receiving a commission of this nature is an honour, since usually only people with international standing in their field are invited to take up such commissions. The benefits of undertaking commissioned work include:

- the kudos of being asked to undertake the work
- a unique opportunity to make a significant contribution of knowledge to the field
- further recognition for your work
- a unique opportunity to have an impact on the world (especially if the work is being commissioned to inform and improve policy and practice)
- personal and professional development
- an opportunity to demonstrate your capabilities and to fulfil job performance criteria.

Commissioned work is not, however, without its challenges. One of the biggest challenges is that often the parameters of the work are specified beforehand by the commissioning organisation or institution, leaving the author with little scope for using their professional discretion in deciding who to collaborate with (in the event of co-authored commissioned work), the content and structure of the work, and how and to whom—if at all—it will be presented (it is not uncommon for a commissioning organisation to place an embargo on pub-lishing the work or at least requiring permission before any part of the work can be published). Ultimately, those who have commissioned the work have the final say on how—and if—the work will be used. These and related challenges are best dealt with preventatively, rather than remedially, such as by:

- *being clear about what is involved in undertaking a commis-sioned work and what is expected of you before accepting an invitation to do it.* In particular, clarify the:

—subject matter

—rationale for writing the work (why has it been commissioned?)

—purpose, aims, and objectives of the work

—intended audience

—how the work will be distributed and its findings disseminated

—how the work will be used

—author rights and responsibilities (including issues of intellectual copyright, author acknowledgement [do not assume that your name will be on the cover], copy-editing resources and production standards, processes for dispute resolution, word limit, and timelines)

—credentials, experience, and reputation of other participating co-authors (where relevant).

- *ascertaining whether you agree generally with the scope of the work, including its purpose, aims, and objectives.* If there is no room for negotiation and you have moral qualms about what is being requested and/or are ideologically opposed to what is being commissioned, DO NOT DO IT; remember: *what can look like a missed opportunity often is not*)

- *clarifying your availability and commitment to undertaking the work.* If you have other pressing commitments that may interfere with your ability to produce the work on time and at the standard expected, or your heart is not in it, you should seriously consider *not* accepting the invitation)

- *having a back-up plan.* In the event that you do find yourself commissioned and engaged in a work that is proving to be problematic, consult immediately with the commissioning body and seek to negotiate a solution to the problems being experienced; due to the mutual vested interests in the work, mutually agreeable solutions can usually be found).

CHALLENGES OF CONVERTING ASSIGNMENTS AND MINOR THESES INTO PUBLICATIONS

Students and colleagues sometimes ask whether an essay, an assignment, or a minor thesis written for the purposes of fulfilling the assessment requirements of a university or professional development course is suitable for publication. The conventional view on this issue is that, in most instances, assignments written for the purposes of assessment are *not* suitable for publication—at least not unless they are substantially revised. The reasoning behind this view is that assignments of this nature (including minor theses) are generally written to demonstrate student learning rather than 'to make a significant contribution of knowledge to the field'.

In contradistinction to the nature and purpose of academic and professional writing, it is commonly assumed and understood that coursework assignments are:

- generally written for the purposes of enabling the writer to demonstrate to a teacher/examiner their *intellectual development*, not to participate in ongoing professional conversations on a given topic
- intended for only *one* reader (the teacher) or in the case of minor theses (one or two examiners), not a broader professional audience
- designed to assist in the development of writing skills for future academic and professional writing, not to expand interest in a subject and provide scholarly leadership in the field
- not readily transferable to suit the purposes of another context (such as publication), at least not without modification.

These assumptions, however, are not necessarily well founded. Students can and do write leading edge essays and minor theses, and these should not be dismissed as being unsuitable for publication *just because* they have been written for the purposes of formal assessment in a university or a professional development course. This is particularly so in the case of assignments that have been written on a 'free topic' and when the writers (often postgraduate students with considerable professional practice experience) have been encouraged to write on a topic relevant to their profession and practice. In some courses, assignments are set precisely for the purposes of intellectual and professional development and are assessed and graded on the basis of whether they meet publication standards and are thus suitable for submission for review and publication in a professional journal.

Each case should be judged on its own individual merits. Whether an assignment, essay, or a minor thesis contains material that is suitable for publication depends on an appraisal of:

- the subject of the essay, assignment, or minor thesis and whether it stands to make a significant contribution of knowledge to the field
- how well the work has been written and whether it complies with the standards expected of writing that is published in professional journals and foundational texts.

Contributions are useful and stand to make a significant contribution of knowledge to the field when:

- they expand on or clarify what others have said
- they offer alternative perspectives
- they make connections with related subjects
- they make a material difference to the status quo
- the new or innovative dimension(s) of the work can be discerned and explained.

Students and academic or professional staff contemplating revising and submitting coursework essays and assignments for publication need to carefully consider the following questions:

1   Does my work stand to make a significant contribution of knowledge to the field and to the 'professional conversations' that are going on? In particular, does the work:
    • expand on or clarify what others have said?
    • offer an alternative perspective to that which is already established in the field?
    • make a connection with other related subjects?
    • prompt a change in policy and/or practice?
    • exhibit the hallmarks of being new or innovative, and can these hallmarks be discerned and explained?
2   Does my work uphold the principles of a 'good' writing style (such as those discussed in Chapter 3) and comply with the standards expected of academic or professional writing?

All writers should, of course, ask these questions, not just novice student-writers. This is because, as Elizabeth Rankin (2001, p. 10) correctly advises:

> As writers our first obligation is to think about what we are contributing to [professional] conversation—what new information, insight, theoretical perspective, argument, application, approach, or deepened understanding we have to share with others in the field.

PREPARING CONFERENCE PAPERS FOR PUBLICATION

Many health professionals and academics prepare papers for presentation at conferences and seminars with the intention of revising them later for publication in a professional journal. A question they often ask is: 'How do I go about revising a conference paper for publication?' The short answer to this question is: *prepare the paper as an article for publication in the first place* and *then* present its key points to a conference audience, not the other way round.

Writing a paper for presentation at a conference with the *intention* of later revising it for publication is a *trap*. Once a paper has been presented at a conference, it is more likely to languish in a file 'waiting' for revision than is a paper that has been prepared adequately from the start for submission to a journal and from which an author has made a presentation. An audience can always read the finer details of what you have written at another time. When presenting a paper, focus on getting a message across: *speak from the head, the heart, and the soul.* Then refer the audience to what you have written and where they can locate it (either now or at some future point in time) so that they might consider and digest the finer points.

If you do fall into the trap of 'presenting now, writing later', the principles of converting an assignment into an article or book chapter apply (see section earlier in this chapter), as do the principles of scholarly writing and writing well as discussed in Chapter 3.

MAKING REVISIONS

No work is complete until it has undergone some revision. Although a normal and necessary part of the writing process, making revisions is not necessarily an easy task. How well you deal with the task of revising your work—and how productive it is in terms of improving the overall quality of your work—will depend as much on your *attitude* toward it as it does on your skill as a writer.

Revising a work is undertaken fundamentally for the purpose of *improving the work*, and it involves rigorous editing that is focused on:

- checking the manuscript for accuracy and clarity
- removing incorrect or unwanted matter
- selecting, rearranging, or rejecting material included in the original draft
- altering or amending material to ensure 'fit' and compliance with the principles of style.

The main difficulty faced by writers when revising their work is deciding *what* to let go—and then, *letting it go*. The trick here is to *allow and retain only those ideas and material that are pertinent, necessary, and 'best adapted' to the survival and success of the work.*

Arguably a greater challenge for writers is when they are required *by others* (often anonymous reviewers) to make major revisions and to redraft large sections of the work. This can be a frustrating and disheartening experience. If, however, the revisions stand to improve the work, then attend to the revisions with diligence and grace. If the revisions requested do not stand to improve the work—or worse, may even undermine its integrity (as can sometimes happen)—this is another matter entirely. Your best option in a situation like this is to not make the revisions requested and to write a carefully considered rejoinder explaining why you have not made the changes requested. Depending on how your rejoinder is received, respond accordingly.

Finally, there is the challenge of deciding *yourself* that major revisions are required. Provided this decision is not driven by a faulty appraisal of the merits and quality of your work, and feedback from others confirms and validates your own appraisal, simply sit down and undertake the revisions.

SPELLING, GRAMMAR, AND OTHER STYLISTIC ISSUES

Many manuscripts 'fail' because the writer has not mastered the fundamentals of writing: *spelling*, *grammar*, and *style*. Unless a writer has competence in these things, it will not be possible to develop competence as a writer, let alone become a 'good' writer. If you feel that your skills in this area need development then you may need to consider undertaking a course, such as:

- an online course on structuring and writing sentences (e.g.,https://natureofwriting.com/courses/sentence-structure/lessons/stylish-sentences-2/topic/stylish-sentences/)
- an in-person adult education course (e.g., through a local adult education centre, technical institute, or university)
- self-directed learning, such as by studying books and manuals on the topics of spelling, grammar, and style; examples of such works include:
  —*The Art of Styling Sentences: 20 patterns for Success* (4th edition) by Longknife & Sullivan (2002; 2012 edition, available as an ePUB)
  —*The Penguin Writer's Manual* by Manser and Curtis (2002; available as an ePUB)
  —*Publication Manual* (7th edition), American Psychological Association (2020).

Another issue requiring attention is that of writers not using the correct spelling, the correct terminology, or the correct words in their work. Spelling and the use of dictionaries are discussed in the 'Choose your words carefully' section in Chapter 3. In the case of the latter, it is good practice to have a small, dedicated table near your writing desk or computer for your dictionary. This will allow easy access to it for checking words and, in turn, will help you to cultivate the habit of checking words regularly.

A final word of warning about spelling: *never* rely on a computer spellchecker to check the spelling in any writing you prepare for publication. They are not foolproof, and you do not have full control over the quality of the dictionary the computer uses for this function. Moreover, a word might be spelled correctly but, embarrassingly, be the wrong word. An example can be found in the use of the word 'public' when writing on public health issues. An inadvertent typographical error could result in the word 'pubic' being used instead, but because of being spelled correctly, is not picked up by a computer spellchecker.

Finally, there is the issue of poor style—both in the structure of the work and in the expression of its content. As the issues of style and structure have already been addressed in Chapter 3 and Chapter 5, just two comments remain to be made here:

- pay attention to the elements and principles of style
- pay attention to the principles of structure.

Writing that is not presented in a clear, direct, simple, coherent, and engaging manner will simply not be read.

BACK-UP COPIES

There has been many a sad story involving writers who have 'lost' their work on account of their computer malfunctioning, being hacked, or being stolen. There is one remedy for this situation: *always keep back-up copies*—both electronic (e.g., external hard drive, USB stick, or secure cloud of internet repository) and hard copies. When closing a file on your computer, always back up and print out a hard copy before shutting down the computer. For large works (such as a book manuscript or major thesis), keep these back-up copies in a safe place (for example, one at home and one at work and even one at a friend's place). This is especially important when you have prepared the final copy of a manuscript. There can be nothing so devastating to a writer than losing a recently completed rigorously edited final copy of a work.

LIFESTYLE AND FINDING A BALANCE

Upon becoming engrossed in a writing career, it can be easy to lose sight of the outside world and to forget that you have other lives—as a partner, friend, parent, sibling, close relative, co-worker, pet owner. It is important not to lose sight of your other lives and remember *to have a life*. Your success as a writer will not mean very much if you—or those close to you—are not around to enjoy it.

Make sure that in addition to making time to write, you also make time to have fun and to sustain and nurture the important relationships in your life. The motivational writer John Kehoe (1998, p. 167) suggests, facetiously, that we should all try to have fun at least three times a day! In response to the question, 'How much time does it take to have fun?', he writes in a more serious tone:

> Sometimes just a few moments. You can have fun in almost any situation. When you are driving to work and enjoying a good song on the radio—that's fun. A joke shared with a fellow employee, a chapter read in a good novel, even a brisk walk in the sunshine or a workout at the gym can be fun.

As an academic, a direct-care provider, or student, adding a writing schedule to your daily activities is likely to make your busy life even busier. It is therefore vital that every effort is made to achieve a balance between work and play. One way of doing this is to designate some 'special time' during each week for engaging in the things that are meaningful and which give rise to a sense of joy.

Include in your writing schedule a 'special time slot' each week and do not allow this time to be violated. Special time must be set aside each week to do such things as: spending time with loved ones, going for walks, cycling or engaging in some other loved physical activity, eating out at a favourite restaurant, watching a favourite television programme, going to a movie, and just generally spending time doing enjoyable things. There is no shame in taking time out; if there is a shame to be had, it is in the fact of *not* taking enough time out to attend to the things that really matter, and which make life meaningful. To those who say that they cannot afford to take time out, my response is: *you cannot afford NOT to take time out.*

CONCLUSION

All writers will encounter certain difficulties during the course of their writing careers. Many of these difficulties are normal and expected, and most can be resolved, such as by using the strategies discussed in this book.

Although writing (and the problems associated with it) can be very challenging, it can also be very rewarding. Most successful writers will concede that, despite the difficulties, it has ultimately all been worth it.

EXERCISES

1   Make a list of problems you have experienced or anticipate experiencing during the course of your writing career.
2   Outline how you dealt with the problems you experienced and whether you were successful in addressing them (what was the outcome?).

3 Outline a plan of how you propose to deal with a problem you anticipate you will experience in the future.
4 Undertake at least one 'free writing' exercise.

NOTE

1 'Free writing' is a technique used by some writers to overcome writer's block. The technique involves unfettered and continuous writing for a set period of time—e.g., around 10–15 minutes— without concerns for spelling, grammar, rhetoric, coherency of ideas, straying off topic, and so forth. It is often used before engaging in formal writing to free up ideas and enable the writer to build unstructured thoughts on a topic without fear of being censured. The technique is not new and its popularisation is believed to date back to Dorothea Brande, an early proponent of the technique who advocated the technique in her book *Becoming a Writer* (1934), which remains in print as a reissued classic (Wikipedia Contributors, 2023). See also 'Freewriting' in Peter Elbow's (1998) classic work *Writing with Power: Techniques for Mastering the Writing Process* (2nd ed., pp. 13–19).

REFERENCES

American Psychological Association. (2020). *Publication manual* (7th ed.). American Psychological Association.

Brande, D. (1934). *Becoming a writer*. Harcourt Brace and Company.

Elbow, P. (1998). *Writing with power: Techniques for mastering the writing process* (2nd ed.). Oxford University Press.

Holmes, M. (1969). *Writing the creative article*. The Writer, Inc.

Kehoe, J. (1998). *Money, success & you*. Zoetic Inc.

Longknife, A., & Sullivan, K. (2002). *The art of styling sentences: 20 patterns for success* (4th ed.). Barron's Educational Series (Available as an ePUB).

Manser, M., & Curtis, S. (2002). *The penguin writer's manual.* Penguin Books (Available as an ePUB).

Maskell, V., & Perry, G. (1999). *Write to publish: Writing feature articles for magazines, newspapers, and corporate and community publications.* Allen & Unwin.

Rankin, E. (2001). *The work of writing: Insights and strategies for academics and professionals.* Jossey-Bass.

Ruggiero, V. (2015). *The art of thinking: A guide to critical and creative thought* (11th ed.). Pearson.

Wikipedia Contributors. (2023, April). *Entry 'free writing'.* Retrieved from https://en.m.wikipedia.org/wiki/Free_writing

Zinsser, W. (2019). *On writing well: The classic guide to writing nonfiction* (30th Anniversary ed.). HarperPerennial.

7 | PROMOTING, MAKING VISIBLE, AND MAXIMISING THE IMPACT OF YOUR WORK

INTRODUCTION

In Chapter 1, it was clarified that the key purpose and primary objectives of healthcare professionals writing for publication is to contribute to and advance the canons of professional knowledge and practice. An additional objective is to share knowledge and vital experiences in a manner that enables others to learn. In order for these objectives to be realised, however, the work must reach and be read by its intended audience. Pathways to an article or book being made visible and having maximum impact in the field does not occur by chance. Rather, it requires *active promotion*.

Once an article, a book chapter, or book is published, the publishers and authors have a mutual interest in ensuring the work reaches its intended audience, achieves its objectives, and has maximum impact in the field. In the case of scientific research, promoting a published report is not merely a matter of personal choice, but an ethical responsibility and increasingly a mandated requirement by funding bodies and other sponsoring institutions (Hardman et al., 2020).

There are various strategies which can be used by authors to promote, make visible, and maximise the impact of their publications. These strategies have been made possible in recent decades due to the unprecedented way in which digital media (i.e., social media, websites, email, SMS, blogs, mobile apps) and other media platforms (television, radio, and newspapers) can be freely accessed and used. Moreover, unlike in the past, when academic authors and clinicians were expected to be 'appropriately self-effacing' when their work was published, today there is an expectation that vital works will be shared as soon as possible. This ethos was paramount during the COVID-19 pandemic, which saw an unprecedented level of unfettered sharing of published research and commentaries— made possible due to major academic publishing houses granting open access to articles addressing issues associated with the COVID-19 pandemic.

Many of the world's top-ranking international publishers of healthcare and health science–related journals (e.g., Elsevier, Cambridge University Press, Oxford University, Sage, Springer, Taylor & Francis/Routledge, Wiley-Blackwell) have explicit guidelines for authors and editors on how to promote their articles and maximise their visibility and impact in the field. These guidelines also clarify the rules and conditions that must be met by authors when sharing their works digitally or by other (e.g., print) media. Depending on the conditions set by a publisher, authors have the option of either making full copies of their articles publicly available which users can download directly, or by conditional requests made available to users for their 'private use only'. In either case, it is incumbent on authors to carefully check the publishers' conditions for using digital and other media platforms before posting information about and promoting their works.

Many academic publishers now have their own in-house publication promotion services, which make available visual abstracts, infographics, and videos (see, for example, Taylor & Francis, 'Promote your article', at https://authorservices.taylorandfrancis.com/research-impact/promote-your-published-article/; and Routledge, 'Promoting your book', at www.routledge.com/our-customers/authors/support-and-services/promoting-your-book). Authors are encouraged to link with these services to help promote their works and increase their downloads and citations.

The various platforms and processes authors might use are briefly outlined under separate subheadings in what follows.

PROFESSIONAL SYMPOSIUMS
Conferences and seminars

A useful and important way to promote your work is through seminar and conference presentations. Performance as a public speaker at conference venues and seminars is an effective way to:

- get valuable feedback on your ideas (audiences are rarely slow or shy in voicing their opinions)
- enable your readers to gain access to you and to feel a sense of connection with a 'real' person and their work (ultimately, it is your readers who are your greatest advertisement, and you should look after them; being accessible is one way of showing them respect and 'looking after them')
- develop a professional network and facilitate the dissemination of the work.

When attending a conference or seminar as a presenter, it is entirely appropriate to:

- present the findings of your work in your paper
- network to foster the promotion of your work by others
- (in the case of books) arrange with your publisher for fliers and possibly some complimentary copies of the work to be distributed to delegates
- promote your work yourself (for example, by holding a book signing session).

Utilisation of scholarship in education and professional practice development

It is important to recognise that teaching and practice can be a valuable source of ideas for research and scholarship, and vice versa. It is not immodest, 'wrong', or inappropriate (provided that there is no conflict of interest, for example, unreasonable financial gain) to:

- list your publications, where relevant, as recommended reading in the educational programmes that you teach or facilitate (in the case of books for which an academic author receives royalties, universities generally require a formal 'Conflict of Interest' declaration to be made and a defence provided of why the author's work rather than a competing title is being prescribed or recommended as a text)
- make your publications available to others such as by ordering them for or placing them on 'closed reserve' in a library
- recommend your work to others for educational and professional development purposes.

Actively promoting your work also provides an opportunity to break the 'politics of envy' that may be operating in your workplace environment (see reference to Susan Mitchell in Chapter 4). Lead by example and praise the work of your colleagues by:

- commending and recommending their publications to others
- referring to their publications in your own work
- including their publications in your recommended readings lists for students

- acknowledging the kudos their successful publications are bringing to your organisation and to those associated with it
- giving them positive feedback (everyone loves positive feedback!).

DIGITAL PLATFORMS AND COLLABORATION NETWORKS

In the intervening decades since this book was first published, the publication landscape and the means by which publications can be promoted and their impact maximised have changed dramatically. In the past, authors had to rely on traditional advertising by their publishers (such as via paper fliers, mailout journals, and book catalogues), and themselves (e.g., by speaking at professional forums such as conferences, seminars, and workshops) to promote their work. Today, thanks to the internet and the many digital platforms it supports, opportunities now abound for both authors and publishers to promote, make visible, and maximise the impact of their publications both within and outside their discipline fields.

Popular professional online digital platforms of relevance to authors include (but are not limited to): ORCID, Research-Gate, Kudos, LinkedIn, Google Scholar Alerts and Google Scholar Profile, and institutional (e.g., university) repositories. Information about these platforms are briefly outlined under separate subheadings in what follows.

ORCID

ORCID (an acronym for **O**pen **R**esearcher and **C**ontributor **ID)** is a global, not-for-profit organisation that enables scholars and researchers to engage with each other across disciplines and countries. Scholars and researchers who register with ORCID are assigned a uniquely persistent and trustworthy identifier (an ORCID number) which they can use when engaging in research, scholarship, and innovative activities. According to its webpage, ORCID enables this engagement by providing the following three interrelated services:

1 The ORCID iD—a unique, persistent identifier free of charge to researchers
2 An ORCID record connected to the ORCID iD, and
3 A set of application programming interfaces (APIs), as well as the services and support of communities of practice that enable interoperability between an ORCID record and member organizations so researchers can choose to allow connection of their iD with their affiliations and contributions.

As a non-for-profit organisation, ORCID's activities are sustained by fees from its member organisations, which include research organisations, publishers, funders, and professional associations. Further information about ORCID can be obtained by visiting https://info.orcid.org/what-is-orcid/.

ResearchGate (R^G)

ResearchGate is a free online professional network of scientists and researchers. Its primary purpose is to foster research communities by enabling scientists and researchers to share their knowledge and expertise. When permitted by publisher guidelines, researchers can also share their publications and preprints, which users can either downloaded directly from the platform or request as a copy for 'private use only'. Although only researchers can register, those who are not registered can still browse the site for content and publications, and to ask questions.

To register, researchers must enter their name, a brief profile, and institutional email address, and choose a password. Once registered, they can upload information about their research, publications, and articles for sharing. The site provides data computations of a researcher's overall publications statistics ('Research Interest Score'), which are listed under the following categories: research interest, reads (including full-text reads), citations (of new and upcoming research), recommendations, and h-index excluding self-citations (an h-index is calculated by the number of publications an author has and how often each has been cited. Thus, 20 articles cited 20 times results in an h-index of 20. An h-index of 20 is regarded as 'good', whereas an h-index of 60 is regarded as outstanding).

Information about the position, discipline, and country of those who have accessed a publications is also available. Further information about R^G can be obtained by visiting https://explore.researchgate.net/).

Kudos

Kudos is an online platform designed to facilitate the communication of scientific research to a global audience, both within and outside the academy. It offers three levels of membership:

- Basic (which is free)
- Premium (for a modest annual fee)
- Research Groups (for an incremental fee tailored to one of three options: a Silver, Gold, or Platinum package).

The higher-level Silver, Gold, or Platinum packages offer additional resources aimed at enhancing global reach and influence. Common to all levels, however, is the sharing and tracking of research across multiple platforms. Further information about Kudos can be obtained by visiting: https://info.growkudos.com/landing/researchers.

LinkedIn

LinkedIn is an online professional network that links millions of members across more than 200 countries and territories. It provides members with the opportunity to share their professional profiles and to post information about their work—including research, publications, and affiliations. Further information about LinkedIn can be found by visiting https://about.linkedin.com/.

Google Scholar alerts and Google Scholar profile

Google Scholar alerts is an online content detection and notification platform that enables users to search for and be alerted to new articles, working papers, books, and other scholarly publications. Google Scholar alerts can be set up to specifically notify a researcher when a new work matching their interests is published.

Researchers can also set up a 'Google Scholar profile', which enables an author to showcase their academic publications. Registration enables authors to track who is citing their work and to compute citation metrics. Further information about Google Scholar alerts and setting up a Google Scholar profile can be obtained by visiting https://scholar.google.com/intl/en/scholar/citations.html.

SOCIAL MEDIA

Social media can be a very successful means of promoting your publications and reaching your target audience. Some have argued that due to its effectiveness in reaching an author's target audience, social media engagement should also be recognised as a form of scholarship and used for assessing academic accomplishment in the health professions (Acquaviva et al., 2020).

Among the most popular platforms available to authors are Facebook, Twitter, Instagram, YouTube, and weblogs (termed 'blogs' for short). If you are unsure about how to use these platforms to promote your work, most academic publishers have guidelines available on their websites clarifying what is permitted and how to use them to ensure you have maximum impact. There is also a range of online courses that can be undertaken on how best to use and get the most out of social media platforms (including what/what not, when, where, and how to post). Such courses can be found by undertaking an internet search using the following key words:

- Facebook for writers/authors
- Instagram for writers/authors
- Twitter for writers/authors
- YouTube for writers/authors
- Blogging for writers/authors.

These courses help to guide learners on how to make the most of their accounts. Of particular note is their emphasis on using the accounts *for their dedicated purpose only*. For example, if you already have an Instagram account for personal social networking, open another account for sharing information about your publishing and other professional activities. Whereas in your personal account, you might post images of your recent holiday and family pets, your 'professional' account would (and should) only include posts about your publications, presentations, and so forth, not your pet dog or favourite café. In order for you and your work to be taken seriously, it is important that your professional account has the appearance of being just that—*professional*, not playful and personal.

A brief description of these digital platforms is as follows:

Facebook—a social networking site that can be set up to enable researchers and scholars to connect, share, and collaborate (for further information, visit www.facebook.com/help/188157731232424/).

Twitter—a social networking site that can be used by researchers and scholars to connect through the exchange of quick and frequent messaging, i.e., using no more than 140 characters, called 'tweets' (for further information, vi sit https://help.twitter.com/).

Instagram—a free photo and video sharing app available on iPhone and Android devices. An account can be set up by researchers and scholars to share information about their work (for further information, vi sit https://help. instagram.com/424737657584573).

YouTube—a free video sharing website. Researchers and scholars can set up accounts to post presentations of their work, for example as a TED talk (**T**echnology, **E**ducation, **D**esign talks are talks that run for less than 18 minutes), or full educational presentation (for further information on how to set up and use a YouTube channel, visit www. youtube.com/).

Blogging—contributing to a blog (short for 'weblog'), which can be an informational website, online newsletter, or journal. Academic blogging can be an effective way to raise the profile of researchers and scholars as experts in the field. Most academic publishing houses have guidelines for authors on how to set up a blog and be an effective academic blogger (see, for example, 'Author Directions: Navigating Your Success in Academic Blogging', by Routledge, available at www.routledge.com/rsc/downloads/ Blogging_SS_r2-web.pdf).

MASS-CIRCULATION MEDIA AND PRESS RELEASES

Undoubtedly, one of the best means of attracting public attention to your work is the mass-circulation media (e.g., print and online newspapers, television, and radio). Most universities and healthcare agencies have a public relations department or unit that can assist and facilitate you in obtaining media attention to your work. These units can assist your publicity agenda by working closely with you to formulate media releases, putting you in contact with journalists, and arranging interviews with either radio or television broadcasters. The advantages of media publicity are that:

- it is free
- it will help spread knowledge of your work and its findings to a broader audience, including the general public
- it brings kudos to your employing institution, to your profession, and to you
- it helps to further the reputation of your department/ university/healthcare agency as a centre of excellence
- it demonstrates the impact of your work (it has been deemed worthy of notice).

There are, however, also a number of disadvantages in getting your work publicised in the mass media. These include:

- the reports may not come out when you want them to
- the reports may not appear where you want them to (they may, for example, appear on page 30 of a newspaper instead of page 1; or they may appear only in regional papers, not in the newspapers that enjoy mass circulation)
- the reports may not be accurate and may contain misleading information or quote you incorrectly
- journalists and broadcasters may only be able to contact you for comment out of hours or during highly inconvenient times, such as very early in the morning or extremely late at night (I have done interviews at 5 a.m. and midnight, on the way to the airport, and in the middle of dinner)
- the publicity you get may be 'bad'
- your privacy may be intruded upon by a public whose interest has been aroused in your work (expect to get

unsolicited phone calls and letters—both good and bad; be also aware of the risk of online abuse and being trolled, especially if your work is of a controversial nature).

To ensure that you get the best out of media publicity of your work, ensure that you:

- *have* a media strategy
- foster a good relationship with the team in your university's or healthcare agency's public relations department/unit (keep them informed, give them timely notice of a pending story, treat them with courtesy and respect, respond quickly to their requests for information and comment)
- foster a good relationship with sympathetic journalists and broadcasters (be available and accessible, respond quickly to their calls, ensure they are briefed well about your work and in a timely manner, always be courteous and professional in your dealings with them, give them 'first option' on doing an exclusive report)
- keep a list and the contact details of possible media outlets relevant to your field
- have something interesting to publicise
- be clear about the message you want to get across in the media
- undergo media training (this can be very helpful if you are likely to be interviewed by radio or television journalists and podcasters/broadcasters).

INSTITUTIONAL AND STAFF PROFILES

Staff profiles—Higher education institutions and healthcare related organisations include web-based profiles of their academic staff and researchers. Staff profiles are a form of 'academic branding', so like any good writing, it is important that they are carefully crafted, accurate, honest, and compelling. The idea is to draw attention to you and your work by highlighting what is worth knowing about you. Staff profiles are an important way for scholars and researchers to get known both within and outside their employing institution. In addition to a short 'bio', scholars and researchers are generally required to provide a longer biography—of several paragraphs—on their institutional webpage. Typically, profiles include a staff member's:

- *full name* (if you have a 'preferred name' that you and those who know you commonly use, *do not use this*; ensure you use the full name that appears on your publications—otherwise, these might be missed or unable to be verified for online detection or audit purposes)
- *academic degrees* (list the type, date, and conferring institution)
- *current position*
- *department or division* in which you are located
- *research interests*
- *awards or distinctions* (e.g., merit awards, prestigious prizes)
- *publications* (with full citation details).

Email signature—depending on your institution's policies (noting that some organisations permit only their own standard branding to be included in staff email signatures), email signatures can be used to include links to and hence promote your most recent publications. Some publishers (e.g., Elsevier, Sage, Taylor & Francis) also provide templates for how best to set up an email signature to promote an author's publications. Some publishers—for example, Taylor & Francis—also enable a 'personal banner' to be created for this purpose (see https://authorservices.taylorandfrancis.com/research-impact/promote-your-published-article/). Before setting up an email link, however, it is important to first check your employer organisation's policy and what is and is not permitted.

Institutional repositories—Institutions such as universities and colleges of higher education have a major role to play in scholarly publishing, which includes maintaining repositories of both published and unpublished research (Slowe, 2018). Such repositories can also help ensure the digital preservation and open availability of research works. Just what publications can be uploaded will depend on the licensing arrangements institutions have with academic publishers and digital platforms. Institutional repositories also enable a researcher's publications to be audited, protected, and kept on the horizon of participatory research and scholarship (Slowe, 2018).

SHARED VOICES—LESSONS FROM HISTORY

As noted earlier, authors in the past were expected to be 'appropriately self-effacing' when their work was published—and it is reasonable to suggest that today, there is a place for appropriate modesty and good manners in the way you go about discussing your achievements. Certainly, boasters can be irritating, and you do not want to put people off *you* and hence your work. But there is no place for side-stepping the responsibility to promote a published work that could influence policy and practice in a manner that would significantly improve the lives and wellbeing of others who are vulnerable.

There are many instructive examples in history where professional jealousies (see comments made by Susan Mitchell in Chapter 4), politics, and restrictions on publishing (especially by clinicians) saw the marginalisation of important works that, had they been widely disseminated (including to the public), promoted, and accepted at the time, could have improved the wellbeing or saved the lives of thousands and even millions of people. To cite just three examples:

- *Puerperal sepsis*—had the observations and reports by Scottish physician Alexander Gordon (1795), American physician and anatomist Oliver Wendell Holmes (1855), and Hungarian physician and scientist Ignaz Philipp Semmelweis (1861) on the possible cause and spread of puerperal sepsis been accepted by the scientific community and medical profession at the time (Semmelweis's recommendations were ignored for 60 years), thousands of women could have been prevented from contracting the disease and dying or having total hysterectomies as a result (Dunn, 2007; Lane et al., 2010; Nuland, 2003).
- *Child abuse*—had the articles on child abuse first published in the *British Medical Journal* (*BMJ*) in the 1860s not been ignored (see BMJ, 1868a, 1868b, 1868c, 1868d, 1868e, 1868f, 1896), the medical profession in common-law countries could have made a major contribution to the prevention and treatment of child abuse *100 years* before it eventually did so (Johnstone, 2023, pp. 284–285).
- *Tuberculosis*—had important early articles on the nature of the tubercule bacillus and possible means of penetrating its outer membrane to allow its effective treatment not been overlooked or treated with disbelief by sections of the medical profession (see Ryan, 1992), not only would a cure for tuberculosis have been found much earlier than it was, but we may possibly even not be facing the new drug-resistant tuberculosis epidemic that we are today.

There are many modern parallels to these historical examples which yield valuable lessons of equal importance about the moral imperatives of promoting vital research and experiences from the field and the dangers of a health issue becoming politicised, deplored, and ultimately dismissed to the detriment of people's health (see, for example, Michael Lewis, *The Premonition: A Pandemic Story* (2021); Merrill Singer, 'The Politics of AIDS' (1994); and Jonathan Quick and Bronwyn Fryer, *The End of Epidemics: The Looming Threat to Humanity and How to Stop It* (2018).

CONCLUSION

It is important that once a work is published, every effort is made to ensure that it becomes known to its target audience and beyond. Often the best way to promote a published work is via professional conferences and seminars, digital and social media, and mass-circulation media, as well as through recommending publications as educational resources in formal education or staff development programmes.

It is generally accepted that the writing process is complete once a manuscript has been *published*. The writing process is never complete, however, until the work has been published, promoted, and translated into practice.

EXERCISES

1 Locate and review your publisher's guidelines for using its author promotion services.
2 Obtain the names and contact details of the staff working in the public relations or media unit in your employing institution.
3 Clarify the process for engaging their assistance when seeking publicity for your work.

4   Source and familiarise yourself with media release kits and tools.
5   Evaluate your need for and undertake a short media training course
6   Undertake an internet search and identify suitable courses that are available on digital media for authors/writers.

REFERENCES

Acquaviva, K. D., Mugele, J., Abadilla, N., Adamson, T., Bernstein, S. L., Bhayani, R. K., . . . & Trudell, A. M. (2020). Documenting social media engagement as scholarship: A new model for assessing academic accomplishment for the health professions. *Journal of Medical Internet Research, 22*(12), e25070.

British Medical Journal. (1868a). *British Medical Journal, 1*(369), 75–78.

British Medical Journal. (1868b). *British Medical Journal, 1*(371), 127–128.

British Medical Journal. (1868c). *British Medical Journal, 1*(373), 175–176.

British Medical Journal. (1868d). *British Medical Journal, 1*(374), 197.

British Medical Journal. (1868e). *British Medical Journal, 1*(377), 276–280.

British Medical Journal. (1868f). *British Medical Journal, 1*(378), 301–302.

British Medical Journal. (1896). Report on the baby farming system and its evils: I.-History. *British Medical Journal, 1*(1834), 489.

Dunn, P. M. (2007). Oliver Wendell Holmes (1809–1894) and his essay on puerperal fever. *Archives of disease in childhood. Fetal and Neonatal Edition, 92*(4), F325.

Gordon, A. (1795). *A treatise on the epidemic puerperal fever in Aberdeen* (G. G. & J. Robinson). Retrieved from https://wellcomecollection.org/works/fhpv49sy

Hardman, T. C., Krentz, A. J., & Wierzbicki, A. S. (2020). Ten tips for promoting your research. *Cardiovascular Endocrinology & Metabolism*, *9*(1), 30–35. DOI: 10.1097/XCE.0000000000000191

Holmes, O. W. (1855). *Puerperal fever, as a private pestilence*. Ticknor and Fields.

Johnstone, M-J. (2023). *Bioethics: A nursing perspective* (8th ed.). Elsevier.

Lane, H. J., Blum, N., & Fee, E. (2010). Oliver Wendell Holmes (1809–1894) and Ignaz Philipp Semmelweis (1818–1865): Preventing the transmission of puerperal fever. *American Journal of Public Health*, *100*(6), 1008–1009. DOI: 10.2105/AJPH.2009.185363

Lewis, M. (2021). *The premonition: A pandemic story*. Allen Lane, an imprint of Penguin Books.

Nuland, S. B. (2003). *The doctors' plague: Germs, childbed fever, and the strange story of Ignac Semmelweis (great discoveries)*. WW Norton & Company.

Quick, J. D., & Fryer, B. (2018). *The end of epidemics: The looming threat to humanity and how to stop it*. St. Martin's Press.

Ryan, F. (1992). *Tuberculosis: The greatest story never told. Swift Publishers*. Bromsgrove.

Semmelweis, I. F. (1861/1983). *Etiology, concept and prophylaxis of childbed fever* (Die Ätiologie, der Begriff und die Prophylaxe des Kindbettfiebers, K.C. Carter, trans.). University of Wisconsin Press (Original work published 1861).

Singer, M. (1994). The politics of AIDS. Introduction. *Social Science & Medicine (1982)*, *38*(10), 1321–1324. DOI: 10.1016/0277–9536(94)90270–4

Slowe, S. (2018). The role of the institution in scholarly publishing. *Emerging Topics in life Sciences*, *2*(6), 751–754. DOI: 10.1042/ETLS20180141

8 | PUBLISHING NORMS AND AUTHOR RESPONSIBILITIES

INTRODUCTION

As with all activities carried out in a professional capacity, there are ethical/moral[1] and legal issues that can arise in the context of writing for publication. It is important, therefore, that you have some knowledge and understanding of your responsibilities and duties as an author, and the reasons why it is imperative to fulfil them.

The publication of peer-reviewed journal articles, book chapters, and books are all accepted hallmarks of the professional, academic, social, and scientific credibility of the health sciences and healthcare professions. Despite it being obvious that authors ought to subscribe to the highest ethical standards of conduct during their writing careers, regrettably there are ongoing issues concerning writers breaching the required ethical standards of writing and publishing. These breaches are problematic in that they risk bringing the author, their profession, their discipline, and their employer organisations into disrepute.

Reviews of the literature have revealed several areas of concern involving breaches of what may be broadly termed 'publishing norms' (also called authorship norms). The most common breaches identified include instances of:

- unfair authorship attribution
- questionable conduct (e.g., exploiting subordinate researchers/co-authors, being disrespectful to co-authors and publishers, being abusive, engaging in slander, promulgating hate speech, 'gatekeeping' and obstructing

DOI: 10.4324/9781003413226-8

academic freedom, and breaching another's copyright and moral copyrights in a work)
- deceptive practices (e.g., falsification, fabrication, and manipulation of data, 'salami slicing' [i.e., splitting a single study and its findings into multiple publications], citation stacking [making inappropriate citations], plagiarism, biased reporting, and unethical conflicts of interest).

(see Gureev et al., 2019; Hosseini & Gordijn, 2020; Kornhaber et al., 2015; Marušić et al., 2011; Tijdink et al., 2014, 2021)

Before discussing these concerns, clarification is required on what are the generally accepted norms of authorship and publishing, and why it is important to respect and uphold them. It is to providing such clarification that the following section now turns.

THE NORMS OF AUTHORSHIP

Norms are a set of shared values of acceptable behaviour that govern everyday actions with the aim of promoting social harmony (FeldmanHall et al., 2018). Social norms and moral norms (which are a subset of social norms) can be both *informal* (based on general understanding) or *codified* (stated in law and codes of conduct).

The theoretical literature on norms (i.e., examining what they are, how they evolve, how they relate to each other, and who are bound by them) is complex and contradictory, and it has yet to find a common language (Legros & Cislaghi, 2020). Nonetheless, three types of norms are recognised:

- regulative norms (which constrain behaviour)
- constitutive norms (which shape interests)
- prescriptive norms (which prescribe what actors ought to do).

(Wikipedia Contributors, 2023)

In the case of publishing norms, all three types apply. And in instances when these norms are breached, they can result in disciplinary action by an employer or—in the case of registered healthcare practitioners—a health practitioner regulation or licensing authority.

Authors need to be aware that academic publishers are committed to and have very clear guidelines on publishing ethics for both authors and editors. An influential agency informing their commitment is the *Committee on Publication Ethics* (COPE), which provides education and support to editors, publishers, universities, research institutes, and all those involved in publication ethics. According to its homepage, a key aim of COPE is:

> to move the culture of publishing towards one where ethical practices become a normal part of the culture itse lf.
> (https://publicationethics.org/oversight)

Authors need to be ever mindful that writing and its publication has the power to challenge and change the status quo. This power, however, can be negative as well as positive, and can have harmful as well as beneficial outcomes. For this reason, writers must remain vigilant and ensure that their writing is morally responsible, and that the power it exerts is morally justified.

When you write, remember always that what you put into print could have a significant impact on the moral interests of others. It is the capacity to significantly affect the moral interests of others that most imposes on writers a moral duty to exercise care in their work and to uphold the most stringent ethical standards both when:

- determining the object or purpose of their writing
- engaging in the process of writing itself.

When developing your writing career and engaging in the writing process, it is imperative that you uphold the agreed ethical and professional conduct standards of your profession. Many of these commonly accepted standards are as relevant to the purposes and processes of professional and academic writing as they are for guiding professional practice. Over and above this, however, there are also fundamental moral norms and standards that apply to authors (and to editors and publishers), as will now be discussed.

Arguably, the most important moral quality an author can exhibit when engaged in the writing process is *integrity* and upholding the four interrelating cardinal virtues of *prudence*, *justice*, *fortitude*, and *temperance*. These four virtues, which derive from the ethical theory of *virtue ethics*, have their origin in Plato's *The Republic* (written circa 375 BCE) (see Part 5, 'Justice in State and Individual'), later expounded by Aristotle in his *Nicomachean Ethics* (written circa 340 BCE). Before discussing these virtues, however, the notion of integrity (regarded also as the cornerstone of academic freedom, to be discussed in Chapter 9) requires brief explanation.

Integrity

Integrity, like courage, is a context-dependent notion (Thejls Ziegler, 2020). Because authors, like politicians, can have influence in the public sphere, their work and character are inextricably linked to questions of integrity.

Healthcare professionals are bound by the codified ethical standards expected of them as professionals. Their moral integrity as professionals can be measured by the extent to which they behave and carry out their responsibilities in accordance with the codified professional ethical standards expected of them. In the case of being authors, their moral integrity can likewise be measured by the extent to which they behave and carry out their responsibilities as authors—not just in accordance with the ethical standards expected of them by their respective professions, but by the moral norms of publishing. At its most basic, therefore, author integrity can be described as moral integrity in the publishing realm as measured by an author's compliance with the moral standards and principles expected of them when writing and publishing a work.

Author integrity, however, is also much more than adhering to moral principles and standards; it is also adherence to the quality and practice of *moral excellence* and to exhibiting conduct that is of an *exceptionally high standard*—that is, a standard that is generally higher than that which would otherwise be expected of others not engaged in a professional writing activity. In short, it is conduct that is 'unimpaired' and ethically sound in every way.

As will be discussed in Chapter 9, author integrity is important because it stands as the cornerstone of academic freedom.

Prudence

To be prudent is to exercise good judgement, to be discreet and cautious in managing one's activities, and to be practical and careful in providing for the future.

During all phases of the writing process, authors must exercise good judgement and be careful, cautious, and discrete in their writing, in deciding the purpose of their writing, in the means they use for obtaining material to inform their writing, and in getting their work published. Authors also need to be practical and manage the writing process to ensure their future success as writers: *what and how you write now could have an important bearing on what, if, and when you will write in the future.*

When engaged in the writing process, ensure that you uphold the following 'golden rules' of author conduct:

- *Authenticity*—ensure that your work builds on and advances a genuine, reliable, and accurate representation of 'the facts' or issues at hand; do not falsify data or exaggerate their significance; avoid taking a 'straw man' position (that is, inventing a problem that does not exist and addressing it in preference to the real issues or arguments held by others).

- *Honesty*—ensure that your writing is genuine, sincere, just, and authentic; do not deliberately mislead your readers, editors, or publishers; do not plagiarise the work of others; take all challenges to your work seriously and respond to them with tolerance, compassion and intelligence, and in an open and informed manner; when in doubt, seek advice.

- *Serving the public interest*—write primarily for the purposes of contributing beneficial knowledge to the field, of demonstrating public accountability and improving the status quo, rather than for self-aggrandisement; remember that writing is a social service—its principal aim is to serve the public interest (that is, the protection of the public and the public's moral goods/benefits, concerns, or interests) and to improve the status quo, not to serve yourself.

Justice

Justice refers to fairness and to the equal distribution of benefits and burdens. During the writing process, writers must ensure that they *deal fairly* with others (their co-authors, editors, publishers, managers, colleagues, other subjects/participants) and must *represent fairly* the issues, ideas, and entities (people, groups, communities, organisations, institutions, nations) they may be writing about. A failure to be just could have harmful and otherwise preventable moral consequences to innocent others, who could be unjustly damaged and even destroyed by the views, revelations, and arguments presented in a writer's publications. A failure to be just could also harm the writer—their professional reputation and career as a writer could be damaged irreparably.

When engaged in the writing process, ensure that you uphold the principles of:

- *Respect*—treat the people, issues, and competing ideas that you are working with in a manner that is honest, authentic, respectful, credible, and free of unwarranted biases and prejudices (noting here, however, that sometimes justice requires 'positive discrimination'—that is, treating entities *unequally* so that the least well off will gain access to an equal share of the benefits that only the most well off enjoy and enjoy exclusively).

- *Privacy and informed consent*—respect your collaborators' prima facie right to privacy and the right to give an informed consent for the use of any personal or private material that you may wish to quote in your work. (It is generally accepted that people have a prima facie moral right to have control over information about themselves and about who should have access to it and for what purposes—particularly when the information is of a nature that could significantly harm their moral interests; provided there exist no strong moral reasons to override these rights, you have an obligation to respect them.)

- *Distributive justice*—respect the normative conventions of submitting work for publication; ensure only those who make a significant contribution to a work (including yourself) are cited as authors to the work (it is unethical to 'free ride' on the work of others, and do not allow others—including a senior research supervisor or manager—to free ride on your work); do not submit your manuscript to more than one journal at a time (this may unfairly use a journal's limited peer review and editorial resources and compromise its publishing programme in the event that an article accepted for publication is subsequently withdrawn); declare any conflict of interest (particularly when participating in a peer-review process), since this will help to ensure that there is not an unfair distribution of burdens. An unfair distributions of burdens can happen when authors have their manuscripts unfairly rejected by a reviewer who is an open competitor with their work; conversely, an unfair distribution of benefits can occur when a manuscript is unfairly accepted by a reviewer who is an uncritical champion and advocate of their work.

Fortitude

To have fortitude is to have strength and firmness of mind. A distinguishing characteristic and virtue of a good writer is *intellectual rigour*. Intellectual rigour relates to the capacity of a writer to understand, think, and reason in a strictly disciplined, credible, undistracted, and trustworthy way.

Another distinguishing feature of a good writer is *credibility*. The credibility of a writer rests not only on their experience, track record, standing in the field and professionalism, but also on their commitment to the writing process—seeing the project through to the end, contributing to professional conversations, being publicly accountable, being prepared to 'stand up and be counted', being accessible to readers and constituents, and producing work that is believable and which has practical application to solving real world problems.

When engaged in the writing process, the following principles ought to be upheld:

- *Competence*—have the appropriate skills, knowledge, and capability to write well; do not undertake projects that are beyond your ability and which may leave your editors, publishers, and readers feeling as though they have been 'cheated' and let down.

- *Conscientiousness*—be diligent and take painstaking care in researching material for your work and in writing your manuscripts (whether commentaries, opinion pieces, blogs, journal articles, book chapters, books, or reports).

- *Conscience*—have a strong and conscientious sense of 'right' and 'wrong' when thinking about and doing your work; faithfully represent (that is, do not deliberately misinterpret or misrepresent) the views and ideas of others; give appropriate acknowledgement to the work of others when you use it to inform your own work (do not steal their ideas and claim them as your own); do not misrepresent, falsify, or exaggerate the importance of your own work; do not falsify the methods or results of your research; do not obstruct the career development and writing aspirations of others out of fear and envy; do not claim or allow others to claim authorship that is not authentic.

- *Courage*—deal with and act appropriately and effectively in the face of fear, pain, threat, or danger; have the 'courage of your convictions'—act in accordance with your moral values and beliefs, and be willing to 'take a stand', particularly when doing so could prevent otherwise avoidable and foreseeable harms from occurring, or promotes a benefit that would otherwise not be promoted if you did not take a stand; when vulnerable, seek support; if you make a mistake, admit it and apologise.

- *Commitment*—fulfil your obligations and promises even when doing so might sometimes involve curtailing your own interests; keep to the word limit, meet your deadlines, keep to the point; respect and honour the agreements you have entered into, provided this does not require you to breach other important moral standards.

Temperance

To act with temperance is to act with moderation and restraint. It is important that writers control their passions both when dealing with their constituents and when writing. Emotional outbursts and other behaviour that exceeds what is generally regarded as being socially acceptable will serve neither the author nor their work in either the immediate or long term. People may not remember what someone did on a particular occasion, but they will often remember how well or badly they responded.

Temperance should also be exercised in the *act* of writing. This is not to say that writing should be passionless and without life. To the contrary, as discussed in Chapter 5 of this book, writing that is written from the heart and the soul as well as the head can be inspiring and very successful in motivating people to act. It is quite a different matter, however, when writing is obsessive, overzealous, fanatical, or even tyrannical in nature, the consequences of which can be dire. An important historical example of the kind of disastrous consequences that can occur as a result of the catalytic influences of an intemperate publication can be found in the case of Adolf Hitler's fanatical and influential work *Mein Kampf*, in which Hitler expresses his views on the superiority of the Aryan race and the inferiority of the Jews.

Good writing is not merely technically correct or stylistically expert—it is also *morally excellent* in that it serves a morally worthy purpose (a moral end) *and* uses moral processes in achieving its intended purpose (a moral means to an end). Writers who ignore or violate the principles and prescriptions of ethical writing risk harming and bringing into disrepute themselves, their profession, their discipline, and their employer organisations.

BREACHES OF THE NORMS OF AUTHORSHIP

As noted in the opening paragraphs of this chapter, there are regrettable instances of authors breaching the accepted and expected norms and ethical standards of writing and publishing. It is to briefly examining the main areas of concern that the following subsections will now turn.

Authorship misattribution[2]

Authorship misattribution is a leading breach of ethics in publishing domains. Journal editors have long been concerned that the names appearing in the byline of an article are not a true reflection of its authorship (Gureev et al., 2019; Hosseini & Gordijn, 2020; Kornhaber et al., 2015; Marušić et al., 2011; Street et al., 2010). Notable among the practices of concern are inappropriately bestowing 'honorary' authorship (also called gift, guest, ghost, courtesy, or prestige authorship) on a person who has *not* made a significant and substantive contribution to a work; and failing to attribute authorship to a person (e.g., junior researcher or research assistant) who *has* made a significant and substantive contribution to a work. Another practice of concern is the unfair sequencing of contributing authors, with some contributors claiming they should be the lead author of an article when their contribution does not warrant such a placing.

Significantly, a systematic review of English resources published between 1945 and 2018 found that codes of conduct and guidelines had little if any impact on preventing or redressing known instances of authorship misattribution (Hosseini & Gordijn, 2020).

Here two key questions rise: what constitutes 'appropriate' authorship attribution, and why—if at all—is this an important ethical issue for the healthcare professions?

Most leading biomedical and health science journals require compliance with the International Committee of Medical Journal Editors (ICMJE) guidelines, *Recommendations for the Conduct, Reporting, Editing, and Publication of Scholarly Work in Medical Journals* (www.icmje.org). The ICMJE guidelines recommend that authorship be based on the following four criteria (ALL of which must be met by a person claiming or being attributed authorship of a work):

- Substantial contributions to the conception or design of the work or the acquisition, analysis, or interpretation of data for the work
- Drafting the work or revising it critically for important intellectual content
- Final approval of the version to be published
- Agreement to be accountable for all aspects of the work in ensuring that questions related to the accuracy or integrity of any part of the work are appropriately investigated and resolved.
  (International Committee of Medical Journal Editors (ICJME), n.d.)

In addition, the ICMJE guide makes clear that an author 'should be able to identify which co-authors are responsible for specific other parts of the work'. It also clarifies that those who do not meet all four criteria, but who have nonetheless contributed in some way, should be acknowledged, i.e., attributed with 'contributorship'. A notable exception to this is when Artificial Intelligence (AI) is used in crafting a work. In response to growing concerns about the use of AI-Assisted Technology in publishing, in 2023 the ICMJE updated its guidelines to make explicit that:

At submission, the journal should require authors to disclose whether they used artificial intelligence (AI)-assisted technologies (such as Large Language Models [LLMs], chatbots, or image creators) in the production of submitted work. Authors who use such technology should describe, in both the cover letter and the submitted work, how they used it. Chatbots (such as ChatGPT) should not be listed as authors because they cannot be responsible for the accuracy, integrity, and originality of the work, and these responsibilities are required for authorship.

Most university authorship procedures and codes for the responsible conduct of research and the dissemination of research findings require compliance with the ICMJE or similar criteria. Even so, studies suggest that despite not meeting all or even *any* of the ICMJE criteria, undeserving individuals are still being named as authors in the bylines of journal articles. In one systematic review, it was suggested that up to 63% of authors failed to satisfy the ICMJE criteria and that authorship misconduct was around 10 times greater than the 2% prevalence in research misconduct (Marušić et al., 2011; see also Hosseini et al., 2020).

As I have outlined previously (Johnstone, 2017), various reasons have been advanced for why undeserving authorships are bestowed on individuals and why a person might misattribute, misrepresent, misappropriate, distort, falsify, or overstate their own contribution to a work. One reason is that even a gross violation of the ICJME guidelines rarely attracts attention unless it is part of a larger review of research misconduct (despite involving fabrication, falsification, and plagiarism, misattribution tends to be treated as a 'mere misdemeanour' rather than serious academic misconduct) (Street et al., 2010).

A second reason relates to the culture and internal politics of academic units where senior or supervising faculty place more value on the *number* of publications listed in their curriculum vitae, rather than on their *actual substantive contribution to a work*. This stance can be so entrenched in a unit's culture that it is near impossible for junior researchers, faculty subordinates, students, and honest peers to challenge it (Kornhaber et al., 2015). For example, it can be very difficult for a subordinate to challenge a senior colleague who insists on being named the lead author of an article when they have contributed little or nothing to its composition.

A third reason relates to the lack of infrastructure and compliance training in organisations to ensure that author credit is not inappropriately assigned. Thus, faculty and students are either unaware of the guidelines for authorship attribution, are aware but choose to ignore them, or are aware and accept the criteria but interpret them so loosely as to justify attribution even for the smallest activity—e.g., merely reading and approving a manuscript for submission (Hosseini et al., 2020; Kornhaber et al., 2015; Street et al., 2010).

Questionable conduct

Questionable conduct can include a range of unacceptable behaviours ranging from misdemeanours to more serious violations, such as criminal conduct. Notable among the kinds of behaviours that are unacceptable are:

- exploiting subordinate researchers/co-authors
- being disrespectful to co-authors and publishers
- being abusive
- engaging in slander
- promulgating hate speech
- 'gatekeeping' and obstructing academic freedom
- breaching another's copyright and moral copyright in a work.

Publishers have strict policies concerning these behaviours. Some publishing contracts, for example, contain specific clauses obliging authors to:

- behave ethically
- refrain from any acts (including criminal acts) that could bring either the publisher or the published work into disrepute
- treat the publisher, its employees, and other authors with respect and professionalism.

Authors who ignore or breach these provisions risk having their contract terminated. For example, if the contracting publisher learns that an author has engaged in unacceptable conduct such as bullying, using offensive or discriminatory language against the publisher's employees or other authors, or engaging in abusive behaviour toward the publisher and its employees and other authors, the publisher retains the sole discretion to terminate the author's contract.

Deceptive practices

As noted earlier, deceptive practices include the falsification, fabrication, and manipulation of data, 'salami slicing' (i.e., splitting a single study and its findings into multiple publications), citation stacking (making inappropriate citations), plagiarism, biased reporting, and unethical conflicts of interest. These practices are a form of unacceptable conduct, and authors who engage in them thus risk being censured accordingly— for example, by disciplinary action or legal proceedings. Publishers have strict policies about deceptive practices, and it is incumbent on all authors to familiarise themselves with a publisher's author guidelines addressing these issues. If an author is found to have engaged in these practices, they risk having their contract terminated and their work retracted.

The deceptive practice of plagiarism is one of the most common forms of academic misconduct and occurs worldwide. There are, however, misconceptions about what it is, the forms it can take, why it is a serious act of misconduct, and the strategies that can (and should be) used to prevent it (Awasthi, 2019). Accordingly, the nature and impact of plagiarism warrants further consideration here.

Plagiarism

Plagiarism basically involves a writer copying other writers' work or ideas and falsely claiming them as their own. Acts of plagiarism have been described by the International Center for Academic Integrity (ICAI) as encompassing the following five elements:

1 using words, ideas, or work products
2 attributable to another identifiable person or source
3 without attributing the work to the source from which it was obtained
4 in a situation in which there is a legitimate expectation of original authorship
5 in order to obtain some benefit, credit, or gain which need not be monetary.

(https://academicintegrity.org/)

Academic institutions and publishers have strict polices around plagiarism and have sophisticated means (e.g., anti-plagiarism software) for detecting it. The blunt advice to authors is simple: *do not plagiarise the work of others.* Not only is it unethical and deserving of disciplinary action, but in cases where copyright infringements are involved it might also (although not always) invite legal proceedings being launched against the offender. The penalties for committing plagiarism can be dire and can include being dismissed from your position of employment, having your publication openly retracted, and having your career progression stymied.

A related issue that remains controversial in the literature is the notion of 'self-plagiarism' (Andreescu, 2013). This notion is, however, conceptually flawed, philosophically odd, and semantically loose. Plagiarism, as noted previously, is commonly defined in terms of it being the wrongful appropriation of *another author's* work and claiming it as one's own original work.

The notion of 'self-plagiarism' is odd because an author cannot meaningfully 'steal' their own original ideas or 'wrongly appropriate and represent their own original work'. An author may of course breach copyright if this has been assigned or licensed to a publisher, violate an author agreement, 'salami slice' their work, or engage in 'text recycling' (when an author repurposes a text for another publication[3]), but this is not *plagiarism*. Even when copyright has been assigned, publishers generally allow authors some conditional latitude to reproduce/quote their own work. And in the case of text recycling, researchers and authors might need to repeat same material (e.g., background, methodologies, paragraphs that are pertinent to a new work, but which cannot be written in a manner that is sufficiently dissimilar to the original, and so on) (Moskovitz, 2021). An author might also inadvertently fail to disclose to a publisher that they have recycled material from a previous work. However, this can be rectified since—as already noted—publishers generally allow authors some conditional latitude to reproduce/quote their own work, provided it is done so in a transparent way and with appropriate acknowledgement.

It does not make sense to claim an author has 'self-plagiarised' (read 'stolen' or wrongly claimed original authorship of) their *own* work. To label text recycling or other acts of authors using their own work in an honest and transparent way as 'self-plagiarism' is not only conceptually confused but, as Andreescu (2013, p. 796) suggest, an 'innocuous offence' and one that is 'without substance all its own'.

CONCLUSION

The conduct of writing and publishing, like any professional activity, is bound by codified standards of professional ethics and moral norms of authorship and publishing. Writers have an obligation to ensure that they are well informed about these standards and norms, and uphold them when writing and publishing their work. Writers need to be particularly aware of and fulfil their responsibilities and obligations in regard to:

- maintaining their professional and academic integrity as authors
- complying with the ICMJE guidelines on author attribution and 'contributionship'
- abstaining from questionable conduct (which can range from misdemeanours to criminal acts)
- not engaging in and denouncing deceptive practices.

Before submitting a work for publication, authors have a responsibility to check and confirm that they have followed the publisher's ethics guidelines for authors. Issues to check for include—but are not limited to—the following:

1 All authors listed in the byline of a manuscript meet the ICMJE criteria for authorship and that appropriate acknowledgement to those who have contributed to the manuscript have been made (listings should reflect the level of contribution made, not the seniority of the contributor).
2 Declare to the journal to which you are submitting your manuscript that it is not published elsewhere

and that you have not submitted it at the same time to another competing journal.

3 Declare truthfully any conflict of interests (what constitutes a conflict of interest is usually defined and can be found in an institution's research ethics guidelines).

4 Where relevant, include a funding statement (i.e., identify the source of any research funding, scholarship funding, sponsorship, and the like).

5 Where relevant, confirm and provide evidence that ethics approval has been granted for the study being reported (note, some journals require a scanned copy of the ethics approval documentation, including the approval reference number recorded by the approving institutional research ethics committee).

6 In works involving reports of responses by participants, provide confirmation that informed consent was obtained, and their other rights (e.g., to privacy and confidentiality, harm minimisation) were respected.

7 Check carefully for any biases and comply with guidelines for accurate reporting of the research.

8 Provide details of any limitations or weaknesses of the study or report.

9 Inform the journal immediately of any errors that might be found after the manuscript has been submitted or published (this will enable the editors to either correct, retract, or publish an erratum notice about the article, whichever is necessary).

10 Complete a copyright agreement (this is usually done online and is part of the submission process).

EXERCISES

1 Discuss with a colleague or co-author the norms of authorship and the ways in which these might be upheld in practice.

2 Access the International Committee of Medical Journal Editors (ICMJE) guidelines, *Recommendations for the Conduct, Reporting, Editing, and Publication of Scholarly Work in Medical Journals* (www.icmje. org), and familiarise yourself with the four criteria of authorship attribution.

3 Select a journal to which you intended submitting a publication and access its ethics guidelines for authors.

NOTES

1 There is no philosophically significant difference in meaning between the terms 'ethical' and 'moral', and thus they are used interchangeably in this chapter. For further information on their etymology and use in moral philosophy and healthcare ethics discourse, see discussion under the subheading 'The importance of understanding ethics terms and concepts' and 'Understanding moral language' in Johnstone (2023, pp. 10–15).

2 Subsections from this discussion have been reprinted from Johnstone (2017), which has been adapted for inclusion in this chapter. Reprinted with permission ANMF ©2017.

3 Text recycling is defined by Moskovitz (2021, p. 371) as

> the reuse of textual material (prose, visuals, or equations) in a new document where (1) the material in the new document is identical to that of the source (or substantively equivalent in both form and content), (2) the material is not presented in the new document as a quotation (via quotation marks or block indentation), and (3) at least one author of the new documents is also the author of the prior document.

REFERENCES

Andreescu, L. (2013). Self-plagiarism in academic publishing: The anatomy of a misnomer. *Science and Engineering Ethics, 19,* 775–797.

Awasthi, S. (2019). Plagiarism and academic misconduct: A systematic review. *DESIDOC Journal of Library & Information Technology, 39*(2).

FeldmanHall, O., Son, J. Y., & Heffner, J. (2018). Norms and the flexibility of moral action. *Personality Neuroscience, 1,* e15.

Gureev, V. N., Lakizo, I. G., & Mazov, N. A. (2019). Unethical authorship in scientific publications (a review of the problem). *Scientific and Technical Information Processing, 46,* 219–232.

Hosseini, M., & Gordijn, B. (2020). A review of the literature on ethical issues related to scientific authorship. *Accountability in Research, 27*(5), 284–324. DOI: 10.1080/08989621.2020.1750957

International Committee of Medical Journal Editors (ICJME). (n.d.). *Defining the role of authors and contributors.* Retrieved from www.icmje.org/recommendations/browse/roles-and-responsibilities/defining-the-role-of-authors-and-contributors.html

Johnstone, M. J. (2017). Honesty and integrity in authorship attribution. *Australian Nursing and Midwifery Journal, 24*(10), 30.

Johnstone, M. J. (2023). *Bioethics: A nursing perspective* (8th ed.). Elsevier Australia.

Kornhaber, R. A., McLean, L. M., & Baber, R. J. (2015). Ongoing ethical issues concerning authorship in biomedical journals: An integrative review. *International Journal of Nanomedicine, 10,* 4837–4846.

Legros, S., & Cislaghi, B. (2020). Mapping the social-norms literature: An overview of reviews. *Perspectives on Psychological Science, 15*(1), 62–80.

Marušić, A., Bošnjak, L., & Jerončić, A. (2011). A systematic review of research on the meaning, ethics and practices of authorship across scholarly disciplines. *PLoS ONE, 6*(9), e23477. DOI: 10.1371/journal.pone.0023477

Moskovitz, C. (2021). Standardizing terminology for text recycling in research writing. *Learned Publishing, 34*, 370–378. DOI: 10.1002/leap.1372

Street, J. M., Rogers, W. A., Israel, M., & Braunack-Mayer, A. U. J. (2010). Credit where credit is due? Regulation, research integrity and the attribution of authorship in the health sciences. *Social Science & Medicine, 70*, 1458–1465.

Thejls Ziegler, M. (2020). Moral integrity: Challenges of defining a shapeless concept. *Business and Professional Ethics Journal, 39*(3), 347–364.

Tijdink, J. K., Horbach, S. P., Nuijten, M. B., & O'Neill, G. (2021). Towards a research agenda for promoting responsible research practices. *Journal of Empirical Research on Human Research Ethics, 16*(4), 450–460.

Tijdink, J. K., Verbeke, R., & Smulders, Y. M. (2014). Publication pressure and scientific misconduct in medical scientists. *Journal of Empirical Research on Human Research Ethics, 9*(5), 64–71.

Wikipedia Contributors. (2023, March 30). Social norm. *Wikipedia, The Free Encyclopedia*. Retrieved from https://en.wikipedia.org/w/index.php?title=Social_norm&oldid=1147338967

9 | ACADEMIC FREEDOM, COPYRIGHT, AND AUTHOR RIGHTS

INTRODUCTION

As well as having responsibilities and obligations, authors have rights. Of particular note, are their rights to:

- academic freedom
- copyrights in their work (copyright)
- moral rights in their work (moral copyright)
- not to be defamed.

Just what these rights entail require clarification and are discussed under separate following subheadings.

ACADEMIC FREEDOM

One of the most important rights an author has is the right to *academic freedom* (also referred to as *intellectual liberty*), regarded as being part of a wider set of complementary human rights such as those linked to *freedom of speech* (Karran, 2009) and *civil liberty* (Fernando, 1989). As I have contended elsewhere (Johnstone, 2012, p. 107) academic freedom is generally regarded as being of critical importance to the development, improved understanding, dissemination, and application of new scientific and social knowledge, which is of benefit to society and the common good (see Altbach, 2001; Golhasany & Harvey, 2022; Karran, 2009). Although a contested notion, as I have further contended (Johnstone, 2012, p. 107), it is

DOI: 10.4324/9781003413226-9

generally accepted that central to the principle and practice of academic freedom is the idea that scholars should be free to communicate new ideas—no matter how controversial or unpopular—to challenge conventional wisdom and question established orthodoxies without fear of reprisal, censorship, or ideological coercion (Arblaster, 1974; Barrow, 2009; Harvard Law Review Association, 1968; Hunt, 2010; Karran, 2009; Sheinin, 1993). Moreover, given the demonstrable benefits of academic freedom (and its counterpart, free speech), it has been contended that academic freedom as such warrants justification as a universal ideal (Karran, 2009).

For the purposes of this discussion, the term academic freedom—as it relates to writing and publication by healthcare professionals—is taken to mean the freedom of clinicians, healthcare researchers, academics and their students in the healthcare disciplines, and others affiliated with the academic community (including administrators) to be independent in their intellectual thinking, action, and personality, and to 'hold opinions, especially unorthodox opinions, and to advocate them openly and without fear of reprisal' (Arblaster, 1974, p. 14). As such, it encompasses freedom:

- of thought
- of inquiry
- of speech
- of expression
- from the threat and practice of physical and psychological violence
- from oppression and suppression
- from exclusion, marginalisation, and ostracism.

(Sheinin, 1993, pp. 235–236)

In keeping with the views of the English empiricist philosopher and social reformer John Stuart Mill (c. 1806–1873), academic freedom and freedom of thought generally is deemed to be broadly justified on at least two counts: its service to truth, and its service to utility or the common good in regard to the progress of humanity (Johnstone, 2012, p. 108—with reference to Barrow, 2009, p. 188). Declarations (e.g., *The Lima Declaration on Academic Freedom and Autonomy of Institutions of Higher Education* (Fernando, 1989) and more contemporary works (e.g., Karran, 2009) have affirmed this justification.

The suggestion that their work could be the subject of interference or restraint from others, or that the knowledge they wish to mobilise could be restricted in some way, might be a surprise to some authors. Nonetheless, academic freedom has increasingly come under threat worldwide, with academics and students (e.g., especially those critical of government policies) facing disparagement of their research, character assassination, being trolled on social media, and being dismissed from their tenure for speaking out and challenging the status quo (Pils & Svensson, 2019).

Paradoxically, academic freedom has also come under threat due to what Golhasany and Harvey (2022) have termed 'the impact agenda' whereby researchers and scholars, faced with the ever-increasing pressure to 'publish or perish', succumb to institutional pressures for *output* (productivity) at the expense of *knowledge mobilisation*—that is, ensuring their work reaches and is accessible to 'change agents in society, such as policymakers and practitioners' (Golhasany & Harvey, 2022, p. 163).

Academic freedom in writing and publishing is concerned with challenging the status quo and with producing work that is:

- questioning
- critical

- innovative
- experimental.

Academic freedom, however, also comes with responsibility. When expressing academic freedom, the means to achieving those ends must always be *moral*—that is, be done for the *right* reasons, in the *right* way and for the *right* outcome. Thus, the right to academic freedom and the principles underpinning it, does not mean—and was never intended to mean—that an author can make whatever statements or engage in whatever publishing activities they wish, regardless of the consequences.

A poignant example of where unfettered writing is unacceptable and ought to be denounced is when its publication can incite hatred and harm to people. Articles that constitute speech that is harmful (of which hate speech is an example) are not acceptable in any forum and are especially unacceptable when perpetrated by healthcare professionals whose raison d'être is to help—not harm—people. For this reason, what counts as an instance of hate speech, why censoring and denouncing it is not an assault on either academic freedom or freedom of speech, and why it is unacceptable requires some explanation here.

Hate speech[1]
Like many terms used in the political and social sciences, the notion of 'hate speech' is contested and controversial. Nonetheless, there is general agreement that the term hate speech involves an expression (via words, symbols, pictures, gestures, conduct, moving images, etc.) that vilifies and incites prejudice towards and the marginalisation of individuals or groups on the basis of their personal characteristics such as race, ethnicity, religion, and sexual orientation. Hate speech has also been characterised as a form of 'spirit murder' on account of it expressing a profound 'disregard for others whose lives

qualitatively depend on our regard' (Williams, 1991, p. 73). Hate speech commits spirit murder by producing 'a system of formalized distortions of thought' and 'social structures centered on fear and hate' (Williams, 1991, p. 73).

Hate speech expresses much more than mere 'ordinary' dislike or disagreement. It encompasses the expression of 'extreme' detestation, abhorrence, and hatred that fosters a hostile environment manifest as harassment, intimidation, fear, discrimination, and violence towards those targeted.

The harmful effects of hate speech are well documented and supported by empirical evidence, and they thus stand as being much more than a philosophical issue (Gelber & McNamara, 2016). Research has shown, for example, that hate speech can directly harm the physical and mental health of those targeted, assault their dignity and worth as human beings, and—in environments that are hostile to their legitimate vital interests—subordinate and silence them as inferior and threaten their security and capacity to carry out their daily lives without harassment.

Hate speech is harmful in other more general ways as well:

- it persuades onlookers to believe the stereotypes being promulgated and to engage in other harmful conduct with impunity
- it creates a culture and climate in which hate speech acts are normalised, defended, and even justified.

(Gelber & McNamara, 2016)

In democratic jurisdictions around the world, the enactment of hate speech laws have primarily been driven by concerns about the circulation of hate speech by extreme right wing organisations; the documented accounts of 'disturbing levels of racism directed at ethnic minority and Indigenous communities'; and an increase in the prevalence of public acts of homophobic violence against members of the LGBTI (lesbian, gay, bisexual, transgender, and intersex) community (Gelber & McNamara, 2015, pp. 634–635). These concerns have not stopped those opposed to the regulation of hate speech from promoting their fears and fallacious arguments—notably, that such regulation will devastate liberty and the democratic right to free speech (which, incidentally, has *never* been absolute), stifle public debate on controversial issues, suppress the discovery of knowledge and truth, and silence necessary dissent. Australian research, however, suggests that these fears are not only unfounded, but that hate speech laws can have the following positive effects:

- provide a remedy for the individuals and groups who have been personally assaulted or placed at significant risk of prejudice and discrimination by hate speech acts
- proscribe incivility which, rather than silencing discussion on controversial subjects, encourages a more respectful, decent, and constructive discussion of them
- educate the public and influence public behaviour by publicly expressing a commitment to upholding people's dignity
- help to deter people from engaging in harmful behaviours.
    (Gelber & McNamara, 2015, pp. 638–640)

It is acknowledged that hate speech laws might have the unintended consequences of creating 'martyrs' (hate speakers who use the regulatory system to claim they are being unfairly silenced by the state). Even so, the creation of such individuals is rare. Ironically, despite claiming to have been silenced by hate speech laws, dissenters are nonetheless able to 'disseminate [their] views widely through prominent media attention' (Gelber & McNamara, 2015, p. 656).

Healthcare professionals have an obligation to take appropriate action in cases when the health, safety, and care of people are placed at risk by the prejudicial, discriminatory, and/or hateful behaviours of others. This obligation stands not only in clinical practice domains but in the context of writing for publication, as well.

PUBLISHING LAW

Through all stages of the writing process, writers must remain vigilant in regard to the legal dimensions of writing and publishing. They need to make sure that they are well informed about their legal rights and responsibilities and—in the event of a dispute—know where to go to get legal assistance either in the form of advice, mediation or court action.

Publishing law (particularly in the areas of copyright and libel) is an extremely complex and highly specialised area. Although an adequate explanation about all the legal issues relevant to writing and publishing is beyond the scope of this present work, it is worth highlighting a number of general points about:

- the publishing contract and obtaining legal advice
- copyright
- defamation.

Publishing contracts

Academic publishers will issue you with a contract prior to commencing a book or book chapter, or upon accepting a journal article for publication. When issued with such a contract, it is strongly advisable to seek legal advice from a lawyer conversant with publishing law before signing it. Just as you would not sign a contract for building or buying a house without getting legal advice, likewise you should not sign a contract for writing a book or book chapter, or publishing a journal article, without getting legal advice.

General legal advice on a publishing contract for authors can be obtained from a national society of authors, an arts law centre or institute, a university solicitor, or a lawyer in private practice. Societies and author representation organisations generally offer a subsidised contract advice service for members, which is considerably cheaper than engaging a private lawyer. Specialised legal advice on copyright issues can also be obtained generally without charge from a national copyright or licensing council, which exist in most countries.

Most reputable publishers have 'standard' contracts. These contracts do not contain any 'tricks'—but they do not necessarily represent the author's interests, either. There is always room to negotiate the provisions contained in a standard contract to reflect your particular interests and project. Reputable publishers have an interest in securing and retaining a good author, and provided that your requested amendments are not unreasonable, agreement on changes can usually be reached.

When you receive a contract from a publisher there are four golden rules:

- read it VERY CAREFULLY and identify any provisions within it that you find unsatisfactory
- make sure that it protects both your *pecuniary interests* as well as your *moral rights*
- DO NOT SIGN THE CONTRACT until you have *read it thoroughly*, have *received legal advice* and then *reached an agreement with the publisher* to amend any provisions you find unsatisfactory
- ensure you return the contract in a timely manner (if, because of waiting on legal advice or some other reason, you cannot meet the timeline specified by the publisher for returning the signed contract, formally request an extension to the timeline).

Copyright

A critical issue of mutual interest to authors, editors, and publishers alike—and which is dealt with systematically in all publishing contracts—is the issue of *copyright*. Copyright may be described as

> a type of intellectual property that gives its owner the exclusive right to copy, distribute, adapt, display, and perform a creative work, usually for a limited time. The creative work may be in a literary, artistic, educational, or musical form.
> (Wikipedia Contributors, 2023)

It is important for authors to understand that while copyright protects the *original expression of an idea* as exhibited in a creative work, *it does not protect the idea itself.* Neither does it protect information, styles or techniques, names, titles, or slogans (Australian Copyright Council, 2022a, p. 1). Moreover, there are activities that do not constitute an infringement of copyright. For example, copyrights may be limited on the basis of public interest and fair dealing considerations (Australian Copyright Council, 2022a; Wikipedia Contributors, 2023).

In regard to 'fair dealing' considerations, be mindful that these only hold if the copyright material being reproduced falls within the exceptions provided in law. In some jurisdictions (e.g., Australia), merely 'thinking' your use of copyrighted material is 'fair' or that 'you are not making a profit' will not count as legitimate exceptions (Australian Copyright Council, 2020). Moreover, while normative limits on word counts or the percentage of material reproduced in, for example, research is generally accepted, this may ultimately depend on the quality and substantiveness of what has been quoted or reproduced, not the number of words or percentile of what has been quoted. The guiding principle on this issue is clear: *if in doubt, check* whether permissions are required, and make every effort to obtain them.

Moral copyrights

Individual creators have what are called 'moral rights' in a work. These rights hold regardless of whether a creator owns copyright (e.g., has assigned them to a publisher). Moral copyrights are the rights to:

- be attributed as the creator of the work
- take action if their work is falsely attributed as being the work of someone else or is altered by someone else but attributed as if it were unaltered
- take action if their work is distorted or treated in a way that is prejudicial to their honour or reputation.

(Australian Copyright Council, 2022a, p. 8)

Contrary to what some authors believe, provided a work is a creator's 'own' and not copied from someone else's work, copyright in the work is free and *automatic*—and it is therefore not essential for a work to carry the © symbol (Australian Copyright Council, 2022a). Inclusion of the sign may, however, be helpful in reminding people that a work is protected by copyright and that permissions may be required to reproduce parts or all of it.

Depending on the nature of the work, copyright usually lasts for the length of the creator's life plus 50–70 years (Australian Copyright Council, 2022a). The duration of copyright, however, varies from country to country. In Australian jurisdictions, for example, copyright generally lasts for the life of the relevant creator plus 50 years; in the UK and USA, copyright generally lasts for the life of the relevant creator plus 70 years (Australian Copyright Council, 2022a).

For further information about copyright, exceptions to its protections (including fair dealing), and what constitutes infringement, authors are advised to access the relevant information sheets and publications from their national copyright council or arts law institute.

Retaining, licensing, and assigning copyright

At the heart of the copyright issue for authors is whether to and how to:

- retain exclusive copyright in their works
- 'lend' (license) the copyright in their works to others while retaining some rights to deal with the work
- 'sell' (assign) the copyright in their works to others and transfer all rights to the new owner.

The principal means by which copyrights in a work are distributed is via the legal contract (other means can include a written agreement, for example, as in the case of collaborating authors). When assigning or licensing their copyrights to a publisher, an author or creator of a work effectively relinquishes their otherwise exclusive rights to:

- reproduce the material (e.g. by photocopying it, copying it by hand, reciting it onto an audiotape, or scanning it onto a computer disk)
- make the material public for the first time
- recite or perform the material in public
- communicate the material to the public using any form of technology (e.g. via television or the internet)
- make a translation, a dramatised version or a picturised version (for example, a cartoon).

(Australian Copyright Council, 2022b, p. 2)

Most publishers insist on authors *assigning* their copyrights to them. Author groups (e.g., the Australian Society of Authors and the UK-based Society of Authors), however, generally advise authors only to *license* their works. This is because once the copyright in a work has been assigned, an author generally loses all the previously discussed entitlements, or at least may find them severely limited; likewise in the case of copyright being licensed, although to a lesser degree. In either case, it is critical that the conditions under which any or all of the rights might be restricted are *clearly specified* in the contract. For example, an author may assign all rights to a publisher, yet retain the right, on the condition of agreeing to give 'advice' to the publisher, to speak publicly about the work—including reciting excerpts from it—for the purposes of promoting and publicising it.

When negotiating a contract, seek legal advice on the options you may have to limit the rights you are licensing or assigning to a publisher such as by specifying:

- the intended use of the work
- the circumstances under which further negotiation must be entered into (such as for a proposed electronic version or 'e-publication' of the work)
- the period of time for which use is granted (in any event, most book contracts have a sunset clause whereby all rights in a work revert back to the author in the event of the work going out of print or the publisher terminating the contract)
- territory where the work can be published (for example, the publisher should make clear what their intentions are of reproducing translations of the work for sale in overseas markets)
- other imposed conditions (for example, specifying that your name must appear on the cover, that the work cannot be used until consultancy fees have been paid, etc.).

(see also Australian Copyright Council, 2022b, p. 2)

Copyright permission

Owners of copyright have the exclusive right to use copyright work in a variety of ways. This means that unless exceptions apply as provided for by a jurisdiction's copyright act, no part of a publication 'may be produced or communicated to the public without the prior written permission of the publisher' (Australian Copyright Council, 2022b, p. 5). Here, the demand to obtain permission to use copyright material (which, in essence, is a kind of 'property') is much like having to get permission to walk across someone else's land or enter someone else's property for some purpose.

Failure to obtain permission to use copyright material is normally regarded as an infringement of copyright and may be actionable in law unless copying falls under the 'fair dealing' provisions as set out respectively in a country's copyright act.

When quoting copyright material in your work, ensure that you:

- give due and proper acknowledgement to the copyright holder
- do not falsely attribute the work as being the work of someone else (including your own)
- do not distort or treat the material in a way that is prejudicial to the author's reputation
- obtain copyright permission to use quotes that are 'substantial' (either in quantity or quality).
    (Australian Copyright Council, 2022a, 2022b, 2019)

Disputes about copyright

Sometimes there may be a dispute over who, in fact, holds copyright in a work. In the case of collaborative or commissioned works, ensure that an author agreement is in place in which the intellectual copyright entitlements of all co-participating entities have been clarified and agreed to beforehand.

There are three ways of dealing with copyright disputes:

- anticipate that it may occur and take appropriate steps to prevent it
- seek to have the matter resolved by mediation
- seek legal redress in a court of law.

Sometimes an author needs to decide whether resorting to legal action over a copyright dispute is 'worth it', noting the legal action can be costly and stressful. An author might decide that the matter is relatively trivial and thus 'let it go'.

Contractual obligations

All standard publishing contracts contain clauses and provisions covering copyright issues. These are commonly situated under subheadings, such as:

- Copyright, or Rights
- Auxiliary Material, Permissions and Index, or Delivery of Work and Ancillary Materials
- Commissioned Material
- Warranties.

Included under these clauses are the following worded provisions requiring the author to, among other things, confirm that the:

- Author grants the publishers, for the legal period of copyright, the right and license to publish the work
- the work is an original work and does not infringe any existing copyright or any other right
- the author has the full power and authority to enter into the agreement and to grant the rights they consent to grant in the contract.

Defamation

Just as authors have a responsibility not to defame others, they also have a right *not to be defamed*. To defame someone is to engage in actions that cause serious harm to their good name and reputation in the eyes of reasonable members of the community, or to make them shun, ridicule, or avoid them

(Arts Law Center, 2023; Law, 2022). Defamatory actions can occur in writing, pictures, film, radio and television broadcasts, public performances of plays, and statements made on the internet (Law, 2022). They can also involve gestures.

When someone has been defamed, the law of defamation (sometimes called slander or libel) aims to

> balance the right of free speech in a community with the right to be protected from an attack on an individual's reputation in that community.
>
> (Arts Law Center, 2023, p. 1)

It is important for authors to know that legal definitions of defamation vary across jurisdictions and countries, as do the legal remedies that may be applied when legal action is taken. Thus, authors would be wise to check what constitutes defamation in their jurisdiction, what defences might be relevant when publishing a work (see Arts Law Center, 2023), and before warranting to a publisher that the work does not contain any libellous, defamatory, obscene, or unlawful material that could result in legal action.

Authors can be defamed by material being published that is damaging to their reputation or good standing (authors can also defame others in the same way). When someone is defamed, they have the option of taking legal action and suing for compensation for the injury and harm caused to their reputation. It is important to be aware that a person can be defamed not only when they are identified by name, but also if they are identified by nicknames or pseudonyms, or by innuendo. Furthermore, even if the publisher of defamatory material can show that any defamatory content was not intended, this would still not matter as a matter of law (Arts Law Center, 2023).

Defending a defamation claim can be a difficult and expensive process for the defendant. Nevertheless, as identified by the Arts Law Center (2023), there are several grounds upon which the publication of defamatory material can be defended successfully:

1 *Honest opinion* (which co-exists with the defence of fair comment): this rests on proving the comment was an expression of opinion, not fact; is a matter of public interest; is based on 'proper material'; is contained in public documents; is based on widely known facts.

2 *Justification/truth*: it can be proved that the material published is 'true in substance or not materially different from the truth'.

3 *Public interest*: if the truth of the allegation can be sustained and the publication of the truth was 'in the public interest' or justified 'for the public benefit'.

4 *Qualified privilege*: as in the case of publication of fair and accurate reports that have been made in good faith and with proper motive—that is, if the material has been published 'in furtherance of a legal, social or moral duty to a person who has a corresponding duty of interest to receive the information' (for example, making fair reports on parliamentary or judicial proceedings).

5 *Absolute privilege*: as in the case of statements made and recorded in the course of parliamentary or judicial proceedings (recall the number of times that politicians challenge their opponents to repeat their defamatory statements made *in* Parliament outside of the Parliament house).

6 *Fair comment*: if the opinions expressed were honestly held, the defamatory statements are based on facts, and/or the facts disclosed are already well known and accepted by the public; this defence is also regarded as 'one of the essential elements that go to make up our freedom of speech' (Lord Denning MR, quoted in Watterson, 1995, p. 41).

Another forgotten ground upon which a claim of defamation can be defended is *consent* (Long, 2014). When it can be shown that the plaintiff assented and authorised the publication of the material complained of, then publication of the information is not defamation.

There are two main reasons why a plaintiff might take legal action for defamation:

- to restore their reputation (that is, 'to clear one's name') insofar as this is possible
- to receive compensation for the injuries or harm done to their reputation, career, or prosperity.

The outcome will depend on how successfully the respective defences outlined here can be made.

CONCLUSION

Authors have rights as well as responsibilities. Notable among these are the rights to academic freedom, copyright, and moral copyrights in their works. They also have the right not to be defamed. It is incumbent on all authors to ensure that they are well informed about these rights, as well as their limitations. In particular authors need to be aware of their rights and responsibilities in regard to:

- academic freedom
- academic integrity (and the principles of ethical writing)
- publishing contracts
- copyright/moral copyrights in a work
- defamation.

EXERCISES

1 Undertake an internet search using the key words 'copyright agency', 'copyright licensing agency', or similar, to locate the relevant agency in your country or jurisdiction and access its information on the copyright laws in your jurisdiction.

2 Undertake an internet search using the key words 'arts law centre', 'arts and law institute', or similar, to locate the relevant agency in your country and access its publications on defamation law, copyright law, and other information relevant to authors in your jurisdiction.

3 Undertake an internet search using the key words 'society of authors' or similar, to locate author advocacy organisations in your jurisdiction, and access information on the membership benefits (e.g., advice, discounts, and guides), fees, and other resources they offer with a view to joining the society.

4 Check the author support services of the academic publisher of a journal you intend to submit a manuscript to and locate its guidelines on copyright provisions and permissions requirements.

NOTE

1 The discussion in this section is taken from Johnstone (2016). It has been adapted for inclusion in this chapter. Reprinted with permission ANMF ©2011.

REFERENCES

Altbach, P. G. (2001). Academic freedom: International realities and challenges. *Higher Education*, *41*(1–2), 205–219.

Arblaster, A. (1974). *Academic freedom*. Penguin Education.

Arts Law Center. (2023). *Information sheet: Defamation law.* Retrieved from www.artslaw.com.au/wp-content/uploads/2010/11/Defamation-Law2022.pdf

Australian Copyright Council (ACC). (2019). *Assigning and licensing rights. Information sheet Go24v12.* ACC, Strawberry Hills. Retrieved from www.copyright.org.au/browse/book/ACC-Assigning-&-Licensing-Rights-INFO024

Australian Copyright Council (ACC). (2020). *Fair dealing: what can I use without permission? Information sheet G079v09.* ACC, Strawberry Hills. Retrieved from www.copyright.org.au/browse/book/ACC-Fair-Dealing:-What-Can-I-Use-Without-Permission-INFO079

Australian Copyright Council (ACC). (2022a). *An introduction to copyright in Australia. Fact sheet GO10v21.* Strawberry Hills. Retrieved from www.copyright.org.au/browse/book/ACC-An-Introduction-to-Copyright-in-Australia-INFO010/

Australian Copyright Council (ACC). (2022b). *Writers & copyright. Fact sheet G013v10.* ACC, Strawberry Hills. Retrieved from www.copyright.org.au/browse/book/ACC-Writers-&-Copyright-INFO013/

Barrow, R. (2009). Academic freedom: Its nature, extent and value. *British Journal of Educational Studies, 57*(2), 178–190.

Fernando, L. (1989). The lima declaration on academic freedom and autonomy of institutions of higher education. *Higher Education Policy, Suppl. Access to Higher Education, 2*(1), 49–51. DOI: 10.1057/hep.1989.14

Gelber, K., & McNamara, L. (2015). The effects of civil hate speech laws: Lessons from Australia. *Law & Society Review, 49*(3), 631–664. http://www.jstor.org/stable/43670529

Gelber, K., & McNamara, L. (2016). Evidencing the harms of hate speech. *Social Identities, 22*(3), 324–341.

Golhasany, H., & Harvey, B. (2022). Academic freedom, the impact agenda, and pressures to publish: Understanding the driving forces in higher education. *SN Social Sciences, 2,* 163. DOI: 10.1007/s43545-022-00468-8

Harvard Law Review Association. (1968). Developments in the law: Academic freedom. *Harvard Law Review, 81*, 1045–169.

Hunt, E. (2010). The rights and responsibilities implied by academic freedom. *Personality and Individual Differences, 49*, 264–271.

Johnstone, M. J. (2012). Academic freedom and the obligation to ensure morally responsible scholarship in nursing. *Nursing Inquiry, 19*(2), 107–115.

Johnstone, M. J. (2016). The harms of hate speech. *Australian Nursing and Midwifery Journal, 24*(4), 25.

Karran, T. (2009). Academic freedom: In justification of a universal ideal. *Studies in Higher Education, 34*(3), 263–283. DOI: 10.1080/03075070802597036

Law, J. (Ed.). (2022). Defamation. In *A dictionary of law* (10th ed.). Oxford University Press. Retrieved from https://www-oxfordreference-com, f.deakin.edu.au/view/10.1093/acref/9780192897497.001.0001/acref-9780192897497-e-1061

Long, A. B. (2014). The forgotten role of consent in defamation and employment reference cases. *The Florida Law Review, 66*, 719.

Pils, E., & Svensson, M. (2019, October 7). Academic freedom is under threat around the world—Here's how to defend it. *The Conversation.* Retrieved from https://theconversation.com/academic-freedom-is-under-threat-around-the-world-heres-how-to-defend-it-118220

Sheinin, R. (1993). Academic freedom and integrity and ethics in publishing. *Scholarly Publishing: A Journal for Authors & Publishers, 24*(4), 232–247.

Watterson, R. (1995). Defamation: Defences and remedies. In M. Armstrong, D. Lindsay & R. Watterson (Eds.), *Media law in Australia* (3rd ed., pp. 31–54). Oxford University Press.

Wikipedia Contributors. (2023, June 24). Copyrights. *Wikipedia, The Free Encyclopedia.* Retrieved from https://en.wikipedia.org/wiki/Wikipedia:Copyrights

Williams, P. (1991). *The alchemy of race and rights.* Harvard University Press.

10 | PUBLISHING NORMS IN THE SPOTLIGHT: LESSONS FROM THE COVID-19 PANDEMIC

INTRODUCTION

In 2020, the World Health Organization (WHO) officially declared the outbreak of SARS-CoV-2 (severe acute respiratory syndrome coronavirus, or COVID-19) a pandemic. In the year that followed, the urgent need for information on the virus (its characteristics, how it was spread, and how its progression could be mitigated)—together with its economic and social-cultural impact on individuals, groups, communities, and countries as a whole—saw the rapid review, publication, and dissemination of journal articles and pre-prints. The reports published included observational studies, opinion pieces, commentaries, case studies, letters to the editor, and the outcomes of research investigating the nature and impact of the pandemic (Capodici et al., 2022; Delardas & Giannos, 2022; Rando et al., 2021). It has been estimated that between the years 2020–2021 alone, approximately 870,000 research papers from 198 countries were published on topics related to COVID-19 (Capodici et al., 2022). This compares with just 109,000 articles published on seasonal influenza during the period 2015–2019 (Capodici et al., 2022).

AUTHOR MISCONDUCT

Top journals in the field are credited with having responded quickly and carefully to the pandemic and the associated need for information (Kousha & Thelwall, 2022). In order to

DOI: 10.4324/9781003413226-10

facilitate the quick dissemination and sharing of vital information, some publishers explicitly invited researchers to fast track their peer reviews and to reduce content that was not related to the COVID-19 pandemic (Delardas & Giannos, 2022). In addition, many publishers granted open access to their journal articles specifically addressing issued related to COVID-19 issues, making it easier for researchers to access them in a timely manner.

The pandemic, however, also created unprecedented opportunities for rogue authors and predatory journals to publish dubious reports (Chirico & Bramstedt, 2022; Corinti et al., 2022; Johnstone, 2023; Tijdink et al., 2021). The characteristics of the dubious reports published typically included one or more of the following:

- had not been peer reviewed
- had used 'sock puppetry' (i.e., a false online identity created for the purposes of deception; multiple online accounts or 'puppets' can be created by the same user to dominate online forums and spread fake news)
- were based on incorrect, fake, or fraudulent data ('fake science')
- had been published in journals with no credible ranking or published in 'sham journals' which were blatantly fraudulent
- had been published in a credible journal, only to be later retracted due to being identified by research integrity sleuths as a 'scam/sham' publication (Johnstone, 2023, p. 311).

In their systematic review of biased, wrong, and counterfeited evidence published during the COVID-19 pandemic, Capodici et al. (2022) estimated that the number of articles retracted after the pandemic was three times greater than the number retracted before the pandemic. Others have concurred, with retraction rates during the pandemic estimated to be as high as 26% in some journals (Else & Van Noorden, 2021).

The primary reason cited for journal retractions was *author misconduct* involving the duplication of material, plagiarism, fraud, a lack of transparency, and the absence of consent in studies involving participants (Capodici et al., 2022). Capodici et al. (2022, p. 2) acknowledge that some works were retracted due to genuine errors being made (e.g., mistakes made in the methodology or faulty conclusions being drawn). Other works, however, involved the deliberate and malicious exploitation of opportunities to 'submit papers that were of dubious scientific value, duplicating their submissions to various journals, plagiarizing others works, or plainly tampering data to fit their assumptions' (Capodici et al., 2022, p. 2).

LESSONS LEARNED

The instances of author misconduct that emerged during the COVID-19 pandemic have served to place an instructive spotlight on the norms of publishing, such as those discussed in the previous chapters of this book. The types of misconduct discerned also highlight the scientific and social harms that can occur when dubious works are published, for example, fuelling the community's mistrust of science, inspiring harmful medical conspiracy theories, contributing to the COVID-19 infodemic, undermining public health protective measures (e.g., mask wearing, social distancing, vaccination), and 'normalising' threats to frontline healthcare workers and public health officials (Corinti et al., 2022; Johnstone, 2023; Rando et al., 2021). As Capodici et al. (2022) conclude, the publication of dubious research is 'a menace for the integrity of modern science as well as the wellbeing of the global community'.

Another unexpected outcome of the surge in publications during the pandemic was its impact on publication trends and journal impact factors (IFs). Of particular concern has been the inflation of journal IFs which could falsely elevate a journal's credibility (Delardas & Giannos, 2022; He et al., 2023). In light of this, authors would be wise to doublecheck a journal's overall credibility before either using it as a resource or submitting a manuscript to it for publication.

CONCLUSION

The COVID-19 pandemic has put a timely spotlight on the norms of publishing, highlighting the ways and extent to which they can be breached and the harmful impact breaches can have on the wider community of authors, publishers, and the public. It has also underscored the importance of healthcare professionals upholding the highest standards of ethical conduct and adhering strictly to the norms of publishing when writing for publication. As discussed and concluded in Chapter 8 and Chapter 9 of this book, it is incumbent on all authors to subscribe to and uphold such standards during their writing careers and to remember that the goal of effective writing for publication is to share vital information and experiences so that others may learn. It is also to help and not harm the moral interests of others, including—and perhaps especially—their health and wellbeing.

REFERENCES

Capodici, A., Salussolia, A., Sanmarchi, F., Gori, D., & Golinelli, D. (2022). Biased, wrong and counterfeited evidences published during the COVID-19 pandemic, a systematic review of retracted COVID-19 papers. *Quality & Quantity*, 1–33.

Chirico, F., & Bramstedt, K. A. (2022). Research ethics committees: A forum where scientists, editors, and policymakers can cooperate during pandemics. *Medicine, Science and the Law*, *62*(3), 230–232.

Corinti, F., Pontillo, D., & Giansanti, D. (2022, April). COVID-19 and the infodemic: An overview of the role and impact of social media, the evolution of medical knowledge, and emerging problems. *Healthcare*, *10*(4), 732.

Delardas, O., & Giannos, P. (2022). The Great Inflation: How COVID-19 affected the Journal Impact Factor of high impact medical journals. *Journal of Medical Internet Research*, *24*(12).

Else, H., & Van Noorden, R. (2021). The fight against fake-paper factories that churn out sham science. *Nature*, *591*(7851), 516–520.

He, J., Liu, X., Lu, X., Zhong, M., Jia, C., Lucero-Prisno, D. E., . . . & Li, H. (2023). The impact of COVID-19 on global health journals: An analysis of impact factor and publication trends. *BMJ Global Health*, *8*(4), e011514.

Johnstone, M. J. (2023). *Bioethics: A nursing perspective* (8th ed.). Elsevier Australia.

Kousha, K., & Thelwall, M. (2022). Covid-19 refereeing duration and impact in major medical journals. *Quantitative Science Studies*, *3*(1), 1–17.

Rando, H. M., Boca, S. M., McGowan, L. D. A., Himmelstein, D. S., Robson, M. P., Rubinetti, V., . . . & Gitter, A. (2021, September). An open-publishing response to the COVID-19 infodemic. In *CEUR workshop proceedings* (Vol. 2976, p. 29). NIH Public Access.

Tijdink, J. K., Horbach, S. P., Nuijten, M. B., & O'Neill, G. (2021). Towards a research agenda for promoting responsible research practices. *Journal of Empirical Research on Human Research Ethics*, *16*(4), 450–460.

| INDEX

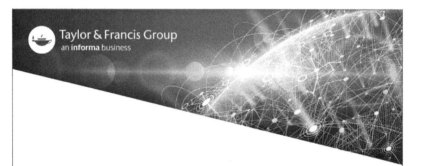